Hoarding, Hoarders and OCD Obsessive Compulsive Disorder Explained.

Symptoms, Causes, Treatments, Signs, Types, Help, Behaviour and Cure all covered.

by

Lindsay Leatherdale

Published by IMB Publishing 2013

Copyright and Trademarks. This publication is Copyright 2013 by IMB Publishing. All products, publications, software and services mentioned and recommended in this publication are protected by trademarks. In such instance, all trademarks & copyright belong to the respective owners.

All rights reserved. No part of this book may be reproduced or transferred in any form or by any means, graphic, electronic, or mechanical, including photocopying, recording, taping, or by any information storage retrieval system, without the written permission of the author. Pictures used in this book are either royalty free pictures bought from stock-photo websites or have the source mentioned underneath the picture.

Disclaimer and Legal Notice. This product is not legal or medical advice and should not be interpreted in that manner. You need to do your own due-diligence to determine if the content of this product is right for you. The author and the affiliates of this product are not liable for any damages or losses associated with the content in this product. While every attempt has been made to verify the information shared in this publication, neither the author nor the affiliates assume any responsibility for errors, omissions or contrary interpretation of the subject matter herein. Any perceived slights to any specific person(s) or organization(s) are purely unintentional.

We have no control over the nature, content and availability of the web sites listed in this book. The inclusion of any web site links does not necessarily imply a recommendation or endorse the views expressed within them. IMB Publishing takes no responsibility for, and will not be liable for, the websites being temporarily unavailable or being removed from the internet. The accuracy and completeness of information provided herein and opinions stated herein are not guaranteed or warranted to produce any particular results, and the advice and strategies, contained herein may not be suitable for every individual. The author shall not be liable for any loss incurred as a consequence of the use and application, directly or indirectly, of any information presented in this work. This publication is designed to provide information in regards to the subject matter covered.

Table of Contents

Acknowledgements 8

Preface 9

Chapter 1: What is OCD? 11

Chapter 2: What is Compulsive Hoarding? 14

Chapter 3: Is There a Connection? 19

Chapter 4: Types of OCD: An Overview 21

Chapter 5: Types of Hoarding: An Overview 24

Chapter 6: Who "Gets" OCD? 31

Chapter 7: Who Hoards? 33

Chapter 8: OCD: In Depth 36

   1) Causes 36

      a) Genetics 36

      b) Brain Abnormalities 37

      c) Neurotransmitter Abnormalities 37

      d) OCD as a Learned Behavior 38

      e) Attempted Suppression of OCD 38

      f) Cognitive Bias 38

      g) Evolution 39

   2) Early Warning Signs 39

   3) Symptoms and Behaviors 39

      a) Fear of Contamination (Cleaning) 40

      b) Checking 40

      c) Counting 42

      d) Ordering and Arranging 42

      e) Repetitive Behaviors 43

    f) Fear of Causing Harm to Others 44

    g) Symmetry.. 45

    h) Sexual Obsessions.. 46

    i) Religious Obsessions... 47

    j) Rituals 47

    k) Other Obsessions and Compulsions 48

Chapter 9: Hoarding In Depth.. 50

  1) Causes.. 50

    a) Environment 50

    b) Genetics.. 50

    c) Brain Abnormalities 51

    d) Psychology 51

  2) Early Warning Signs 53

  3) Symptoms and Behaviors 54

    a) Comorbidity 54

    b) Dangers.. 55

Chapter 10: Crossing the Line: Normalcy versus Disorder 59

Chapter 11: What Other Disorders Are Common with OCD? 61

  1) Major Depressive Disorder 61

  2) Anxiety Disorders... 62

  3) Personality Disorders... 66

  4) Body Dysmorphic Disorder 67

Chapter 12: What Other Disorders Are Common with Compulsive Hoarding? 69

  1) Mood Disorders 69

  2) Anxiety Disorders... 72

- 3) Dementia 75
- 4) Attention Deficit Disorder 78
- 5) Diogenes Syndrome.. 79
- 6) Other Disorders 80

Chapter 13: What You Can Do if Someone You Know has OCD 82
- 1) Who Can Diagnose It? 82
- 2) How is It Diagnosed? 83
- 3) What if Someone is in Denial?.. 84
- 4) For Yourself... 85

Chapter 14: What You Can Do if Someone You Know Hoards 87
- 1) Who Can Diagnose It? 87
- 2) How is Compulsive Hoarding Diagnosed? 88
- 3) What if Someone is in Denial?.. 90
- 4) For Yourself... 91

Chapter 15: Treatments for OCD.. 92
- 1) Medication... 92
- 2) Psychotherapy 93
- 3) Lifestyle Changes 93
- 4) Alternative Medicine 94
- 5) Surgery... 94

Chapter 16: Treatments for Compulsive Hoarding.................................. 96
- 1) Medication... 96
- 2) Psychotherapy 96
- 3) Lifestyle Changes 98
- 4) Alternative Medicine 98

Chapter 17: Treatments for Associated Disorders 100

- 1) Major Depressive Disorder 100
- 2) Bipolar Disorder 103
- 3) Social Anxiety and Social Phobia 106
- 4) Panic Disorder 108
- 5) Generalized Anxiety Disorder 110
- 6) Posttraumatic Stress Disorder 111
- 7) Dependent Personality Disorder 114
- 8) Avoidant Personality Disorder 115
- 9) Body Dysmorphic Disorder 115
- 10) Dementia 116
- 11) Attention Deficit Disorder 116
- 12) Diogenes Syndrome 119

Chapter 18: What Does Future Research Look Like? 123

Chapter 19: A Special Look at Children 125

Chapter 20: Living with a Person with OCD 128

Chapter 21: Living with a Person who Hoards 130

Chapter 22: Working with a Person with OCD 132

Chapter 23: Working with a Person who Hoards 133

Chapter 24: Additional Resources Available 134

- 1) Hoarding 134
- 2) Obsessive Compulsive Disorder 136
- 3) For Children and Teens 136
- 4) For Parents 137
- 5) For Teachers 138
- 6) Treatments 138
- 7) Children of Hoarders 140

    8) Financial Assistance 141

    9) Legal Resources and Employment Assistance 142

Chapter 25: Conclusion 143

Glossary 144

Index 147

Acknowledgements

Thanks to my mum for being such a great mum. Even though she works long hours, she always has time to listen and help me. Her office door is always open to my sibling and I. She is an author herself and she inspired me to write this book.

In addition, my dad always supports mum and us kids in whatever we do. He's always there with an encouraging word and an understanding heart. I especially thank him for taking the time to read this book and offer his valuable suggestions on how to make it better.

Without my brothers and sisters, especially my amazingly, smart, talented, gorgeous twin sister :-), to make me laugh I would never have been able to complete this book.

I also want to thank all the people who generously shared their personal experiences about living with hoarding. I've learned so much from them and appreciate their openness and honesty.

Thanks goes to all the professionals in the field that I spoke to whose experience and knowledge helped me understand hoarding.

Preface

Obsessive Compulsive Disorder (OCD) can affect anyone. Someone you live with or work with may be diagnosed with it, or show traits that make you believe they should be diagnosed with it.

Hoarding behaviors are also common amongst a wide group of people. Whether it's hoarding food, books, animals, or every piece of junk mail, hoarding can be difficult to understand from an outsider's perspective.

The purpose of this book is to help friends and family members understand OCD and hoarding behaviors of their loved ones, so that they can learn to help others, accept them, and know when and where to seek help. Although research is presented in this book, it is explained in its simplest form, so that individuals without psychological training can understand it.

To use this book, it is suggested that you read it in its entirety. However, if you already have a specific interest such as hoarding behaviors, treatment options, or additional resources, the table of contents and index make finding these topics very easy.

In addition, there are notes attached to the end of each chapter, which may include references or the sources of information. This is done to make the chapters easier to read, while still providing the information to further explore additional research.

Also, it's understood that sometimes reading full, bulky paragraphs can become frustrating. To break up the book and make it easier to read, there are symbols scattered throughout that you might bring your attention to. Here's a quick overview:

$Cost: Some treatments and forms of help can be expensive. Look for these icons for ideas regarding price and ways to save money.

Research: Throughout this book, research will be discussed. Some of this information will be scattered right through the book with notes at the end of chapters. Other, specific research will be highlighted with this icon.

Learning: Some concepts need extra attention. This includes vocabulary, a brief history of an issue, or clarification.

Questioning: These are questions to think about regarding individuals that you know who might struggle with the disorder.

Enjoy the book.

Chapter 1: What is OCD?

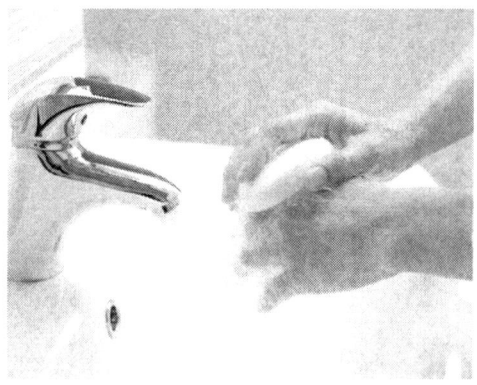

Obsessive Compulsive Disorder (OCD) can be difficult to truly understand. It can also be hard to accurately define without the use of complex psychological terms.

Obsessive compulsive disorder is a mental health problem that includes thoughts and behaviors that are intrusive, redundant, anal, or habitual, usually against the control of the afflicted person, impeding his or her function.

A mild form of OCD may be an individual who must have all the items on their desk in a straight line. This person may show no other signs of OCD, simply this peculiar trait.

A severe form of OCD may be an individual who is injured in a car accident due to the inability to move his vehicle until he has performed his habit of sitting through three red lights. Generally, people with this level of OCD are posing a risk to themselves or others, simply by the lack of control over certain behaviors.

The entertainment industry has discovered the public's fascination with OCD. <u>As Good As It Gets</u>[1], a movie released in 1997,

Chapter 1: What is OCD?

highlighted the characteristics of the disorder in a lighthearted comedy. However, individuals with OCD may not find this movie as humorous, as they relate with the main character.[2]

In addition, Monk[3] was a television show that ran from 2002 to 2009. The show appeared to give OCD a positive spin by showing how a detective can use this disorder to his advantage to solve cases. This show was also considered a comedy.

So why do so many people consider this behavior, which is a recognizable disorder, funny?

Many times these behaviors may seem peculiar to individuals who do not have them. A person who must count the number of times she chews her food on each side of her mouth is seen as "weird". A person who has his closet specifically arranged by the color of the clothes may be considered an "oddball" by his friends. After all, others may simply chew their food or arrange their clothes by the type of clothing, (or just by what fits on a hanger!)

As the name implies, there are two distinct aspects of this disorder: obsession and compulsion. Although it may appear that these terms are similes, they are not in this context.

Obsession generally refers to the intrusive thoughts a person experiences. For example, a person may think "Did I turn the stove off?" even knowing that she did. In order to soothe this thought, she may feel required to turn the stove on and off three times, or six, or twelve.

Compulsion, on the other hand, is the behaviors and actions of the person. Flipping the light switch 21 times before he leaves the room, may be obligatory to a severely OCD man. In some cases, these people become distraught if these actions cannot be finished because they feel something terrible will occur. In some cases, they believe this horror may befall them; in others, it may befall their loved ones.

Chapter 1: What is OCD?

In most individuals with OCD, both of these characteristics are visible and play off of one another. In the stove example, turning the stove knob 12 times is a compulsion, which is "required" to settle the obsession.

? Does this person seem to have repetitive actions that could be considered anal? Is there a struggle with invasive thoughts?

This book will explore the types of OCD, demographics affected, causes, and treatments.
Notes:

1. Sakai, R. & Ziskin, L. (Producers) & Brooks, J. L. (Director). (1997). *As good as it gets* [Motion Picture]. United States: TriStar Pictures.

2. Various observations and interviews.

3. Breckman, A. (Producer). (2002). *Monk* [Television series]. Hollywood: Paramount Pictures.

Chapter 2: What is Compulsive Hoarding?

Chapter 2: What is Compulsive Hoarding?

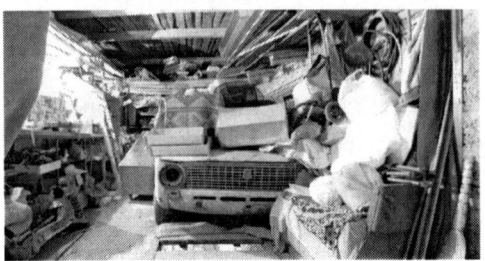

Hoarding might be considered by some to be the act of "collecting" just taken one step too far. However, scientists insist that individuals should not confuse the two. Hoarders are often individuals who keep possessions longer than they should or in greater quantity.

Hoarding is continuing to hold possessions after their intended use has ended. As a disorder, this also usually involves some type of emotional attachment.

This is a very short definition that will be exaggerated later. There are acceptable levels of collecting that do not cross the line into hoarding. Look at the following two examples.

Example One: A man has a fine appreciation for violins and has collected more than 50 throughout the years. He has bought them from thrift stores, auctions, and dealers. He keeps the violins displayed in a multitude of shelves in his library.

Example Two: A mother has one child, a daughter, who she loves dearly. She has kept all of the child's report cards, science fair projects, and homemade holiday cards. Even though she is now a young adult, her mother occasionally reminisces over her daughter's items that remain in a shoebox on the closet's top shelf.

Chapter 2: What is Compulsive Hoarding?

Could these people be considered hoarders by other individuals? Yes. The man does not play the violin; therefore they no longer serve their purpose. The child is now grown and her science fair projects are worthless. But are they truly hoarders? Let's look at a few key characteristics of hoarding.

1) *Practicality: Is it practical for these items to be kept?*

The man's violins offer a decorative display while the child's belongings serve as a preserved memory.

Although these habits may be seen as practical, much of hoarding is not. For example, hoarding every piece of mail received has no practical implications.

2) Feeling: How does the owner feel?

Both individuals feel a sense of pride, one from the objects themselves, the other from what the objects represent. The mother also feels a sense of nostalgia by being able to remember her child's earlier years.

This positive feeling is compared to one of dread that comes from finding the house a mess or that of anxiety from the inability to save the important items or allow others into the home.

3) Placement: Where are the items kept?

The man displayed his violins neatly on shelves while the woman kept these valuables in a box at the top of a closet. Both of these places are neat and structured.

Hoarders may keep so many items that there is no specific place for the possessions to reside. This can be seen in a kitchen with so many food items that there is no counter or seating space. The mail may spill over from the living room into the dining room, bedroom, and kitchen. A person may not be able to find a place to sit because the mail is now residing on multiple chairs and couches.

Chapter 2: What is Compulsive Hoarding?

4) Appearance: How does the person's living or work environment appear?

This goes hand-in-hand with placement. In the woman's case, her living arrangements do not appear any differently than if she did not have the items at all. For the man, his collection may even increase the aesthetics of the house.

However, hoarders who have mail scattered throughout the house greatly decrease the appearance of their space, often increasing the amount of anxiety that they feel. Once the mess extends above a certain point, a person may feel hopeless and unable to conquer it.

5) Disposal: Although this does not directly apply to the two examples given, disposal is the fifth key characteristic of hoarding. If either of these individuals had also had a large pile of junk mail in the living room, could they dispose of it? Most likely. Neither of them seem to have an attachment to mail, only to violins and sentimental documents.

Many true hoarders become greatly distressed when confronted with the possibility of throwing away anything, including junk mail, sugar packets, floppy disks, or candy wrappers. They may feel that these items could still be of use or have an emotional attachment to them.

6) Others: What is the perception of friends and family members? Are there children or others living with a hoarder that are experiencing negative effects? This most notably includes people, but it can also include animals.

As will be discussed later, the effects of hoarding parents on their children have become so apparent, that support groups have been developed specifically for this demographic. Individuals living or working with a hoarder may experience negative consequences that are oblivious to the person who hoards.

Chapter 2: What is Compulsive Hoarding?

7) *Safety:* Does the hoarding endanger the health or safety of themselves or others in the home? Safety risks can include:

- Airborne allergens including dust, mildew, or mold
- Insects including cockroaches, ants, or maggots
- Spiders including black widows
- Falling due to unsafe pathways, (especially true of elderly or handicapped individuals)
- Avalanche of objects that cause bodily harm

It could be argued that safety is the most important aspect of hoarding. Individuals, who are discovered to put their children in danger, risk the children being taken into the government's custody. Eviction may also be a possibility if a landlord discovers physical damage to the residence as a result of hoarding.

❓ How many of these characteristics does the person you know possess?

After reviewing these key characteristics, are the people in the two examples hoarders? No. One is a collector and the other is a sentimental mother. These behaviors are not considered abnormal or require treatment or intervention.

Example Three: An elderly woman worries that she'll starve if a natural disaster were to occur. Therefore, her pantry is full of various foods, which the woman rarely touches.

In this example, the hoarding may create a positive feeling, such as safety, and be in an area that is not cluttered or decreases appearance, such as in a pantry. However, if the food is past its expiration date, and therefore has no practical purpose, this practice could still be considered unhealthy hoarding.

Chapter 2: What is Compulsive Hoarding?

This book will discuss various types of hoarding, the underlying causes, the demographics affected, and the treatments that can be helpful.

Chapter 3: Is There a Connection?

Some may ask why these two topics were combined into a single book. It may appear that these two topics are not at all interrelated. You may know a hoarder who you simply consider to be a "slob" rather than to be suffering from a disorder. Perhaps this person shows no other signs of OCD.

Research regarding hoarding in connection with OCD is a fairly new field.[1] However, evidence has now shown that there is a connection between these two disorders in some cases.

Compulsive hoarding may co-occur in individuals diagnosed with OCD 10 to 30 percent of the time.[1] However, there are several differences between OCD individuals that hoard and those that do not; including genetics, brain abnormalities, and success of treatment.

Research has indicated that treatment may be more difficult to complete for individuals with OCD and hoarding tendencies, rather than OCD alone.[1] This can be disheartening to individuals who wish to overcome these behaviors. There is a chapter dedicated to the treatment of each disorder, seeing as the methods and success rate vary.

Psychologists are beginning to consider hoarding as a separate disorder from OCD, which will be discussed later. However, these two disorders are often interconnected. Therefore, the person you know who struggles with hoarding may also be struggling with OCD and need treatment for both conditions.

Hopefully, the information in this book will lead you to make an informative decision regarding which disorder affects your friend or family member and the steps you can both take to confront it.

Chapter 3: Is There a Connection?

Notes

1. Butcher, J.N., Mineka, S., & Hooley, J. M. (2010). *Abnormal psychology.* (14th ed.). Boston: Allyn & Bacon. pp. 206-216.

Chapter 4: Types of OCD: An Overview

After briefly discussing OCD in chapter one, it may appear that there is only one type of OCD. After all, obsessive compulsive disorder combines obsessive thoughts *and* compulsive behaviors. However, there are levels of extremes and differences in behavior that may not be present in all individuals. This chapter will explore these concepts further.

Combined Obsessive and Compulsive

This is the type of OCD that the majority of this book focuses on. In this type, obsessions and compulsions are both overt. That is, other people around the afflicted person can see the individual's odd behaviors, and are usually aware of some of the obsessive thought processes. This is because the person may vocalize some of these while engaging in the compulsive behavior. For example, a wife may hear her husband ask if he turned the stove off every night prior to checking the stove three times.

Purely Obsessive

There is a type of OCD in which the individual does not appear to have the compulsive behaviors often observed. However, the compulsive behaviors may actually be thought processes and a person may avoid certain situations in order to minimize the probability of the actions occurring.[1]

There are still questions regarding the purely obsessive form of OCD. Some studies have shown that 90 percent, (up to 98 percent if mental rituals are included,) of individuals that seek treatment will have both obsessions and compulsions. However, the incidence of OCD without compulsions may be as high as 55 percent.[2] Other sources state, that between 50 and 60 percent of OCD cases fall in this category.[3]

Chapter 4: Types of OCD: An Overview

The factor that seems to determine treatment is the severity of the condition. Therefore, individuals with the purely obsessive subtype may feel, (due to truth or denial,) that the disorder is manageable and not necessary to treat.

? Does this person discuss thoughts that are constant or cause him great anxiety?

There are several other types that will be discussed in the chapter regarding symptoms and behaviors, rather than in this brief overview. These types include:[2]

- Cleaning
- Constantly checking
- Counting
- Ordering and arranging
- Repetition

As you can see, there are several types of OCD that involve specific behaviors and thought processes. Although an individual may have simply one type or key symptom, such as fear of contamination, some may have several symptoms combined that feed off of one another. The individual with a fear of contamination may also have specific rituals that they practice and they may want everything in a certain order.

These characteristics, as well as several others, will be discussed in depth in the chapter OCD: In Depth. For now, simply understand that OCD does not come in a "one size fits all" style. Different people are afflicted with different hardships.

Chapter 4: Types of OCD: An Overview

Notes:

1. Hyman, B. M., & Pedrick, C. (2005). *The OCD workbook: Your guide to breaking free from obsessive–compulsive disorder* (2nd ed.). Oakland, CA: New Harbinger, pp. 125-126.

2. Butcher, J.N., Mineka, S., & Hooley, J. M. (2010). *Abnormal psychology.* (14th ed.). Boston: Allyn & Bacon. pp. 206-216.

3. Weisman M.M., Bland R.C., Canino G.J., Greenwald S., Hwu H.G., Lee C.K. *et al.* (1994). "The cross national epidemiology of obsessive–compulsive disorder". *Journal of Clinical Psychiatry* **55**: 5–10

Chapter 5: Types of Hoarding: An Overview

Despite what the general population may think, there are actually several types of hoarding. Some of these are conventional, while others may be considered in a new perspective. The following types will be examined: ordinary, animal, trash, digital, book, and information hoarding.

Type One: Ordinary Hoarding

Ordinary hoarding is what most people think of when they imagine compulsive hoarders. These individuals may collect anything including dishes, tools, games, mail, food, or any number of other things.

Although all of these things can pose various risks, food may be the most obvious. Food spoils and can attract various insects and transmit odors or allergens. Causes of hoarding will be discussed later, but many people believe that food hoarding results from a previous exposure to poverty. Research on this topic will be discussed.

Type Two: Animal Hoarding

The notion of "the crazy cat lady" is a common, and crude, stereotype of animal hoarding. Some researchers have claimed that specific conditions must be met for an individual to be considered an animal hoarder. These conditions include[1]:

- Possession of an excessive number of animals
- Inability or unwillingness to provide necessary care of the animals
- Neglect of the animal, which may lead to illness or death
- Negative effects on others including living conditions

Chapter 5: Types of Hoarding: An Overview

In other words, not only does this person possess several animals, (which may or may not be of the same type,) he does not care for them or others. This can be especially difficult if a child is allergic to the animals. For example, an asthmatic child living with animals that increase asthma attacks may be viewed as medical neglect on the part of the parent and result in the parent losing custody of the child.

In addition, animal hoarding may result in severe legal consequences. The American Society for the Prevention of Cruelty to Animals (ASPCA) publishes information on animal hoarding including legal ramifications. Although hoarding legislation has been considered in several states, Hawaii and Illinois are the only states in the United States to have passed such legislation. In Hawaii, animal hoarding is outlawed. In Illinois, convicted animal hoarders must receive counseling. However, all states have laws against animal cruelty, and animal hoarders may be prosecuted under these terms.

In 2011, one case was reported in which more than 400 neglected dogs had to be rescued from a shelter that had inhumane living conditions. In an attempt to "save" dogs that would have otherwise been subject to euthanasia, the shelter had accumulated more dogs than it could care for which resulted in extreme neglect.[2] At least one other case has found 1,000 animals in a person's home.[7]

Type Three: Trash Hoarding

Trash hoarding is also referred to as syllogomania. These individuals literally hoard garbage, which may include trash bags, used candy wrappers, old newspapers, empty soda bottles, etc. As

Chapter 5: Types of Hoarding: An Overview

with hoarding food and animals, this can become very unsanitary and lead to infestation.

This type of hoarding can be a sign of Diogenes syndrome as well as compulsive hoarding. This disorder will be discussed in the comorbidity section.

Type Four: Digital Hoarding

Some may consider that this type of hoarding is not considered "true" hoarding due to its electronic medium. Nevertheless, this has become more of a topic of interest as electronics become more accessible and useful. In addition, the electronic hoarding may "spill over" into the physical world.

Digital hoarding appears to have two subtypes, which can be separate or connected. The first is that of a true electronic medium. For example, an individual may have thousands of emails, photos, temporary files, and documents stored on a computer, many of which are now useless. Some of these items may even be in outdated formats that are no longer accessible, but he is unable to delete them.

The second subtype is of a tangible nature. Although the items may be stored electronically, a person may have acquired hundreds or thousands of hard drives, CDs, or floppy disks. Again, these may be in obsolete formats. These devices may cause drastic clutter, as seen in other forms of hoarding.

Effects of digital hoarding can vary and include emotional distress when faced with the challenge of deleting items, slower computer processing, and an inability to receive e-mail due to lack of virtual memory.[3,4]

Chapter 5: Types of Hoarding: An Overview

There are now companies that specialize in helping individuals clean their computers' hard drives. This could be as easy as running a brief software scan or as difficult as helping a person look through each document, photograph, and webpage.

Type Five: Book Hoarding

Book hoarding is also known as bibliomania. This is not to be confused with a person who simply loves to read, or someone who collects books of a specific age, rarity, or author. Instead, it is a disorder in which a person's social functioning or health is impaired. This may include buying multiple copies of the same book or buying so many books that there will be no way to enjoy them all.

This type of hoarding may follow the same principles as an ordinary hoarder in that the clutter is so intense that it poses physical danger. Books may be piled on furniture, on the floor, or even in beds and hallways. In addition, this type of hoarding may keep a person from even letting someone in the house to make necessary repairs due to the shame of the living conditions.[5]

Type Six: Information Hoarding

Information hoarding is a debatable topic and the information changes with various sources. One researcher reports that information hoarding may fall into three categories: those related to memory, self-sought information, and general information.[6] Information related to memory may include old calendars or other items that remind individuals of previous events. Self-sought information is specific to individuals that feel a specific topic should be researched. For example, a person may want to choose the correct therapist and spend days or weeks looking at hundreds

Chapter 5: Types of Hoarding: An Overview

of documents regarding therapists from their city. Although they may believe this is simply to choose the right person, this becomes cognitive overload and is more information than they truly needed. General information is that which is read but is not necessary at the time including flyers, menus, or labels. Although some of this information may be beneficial, it may also provide more anxiety than assistance.

This could be tangible in post-it notes, memos, and notebook pads, digital in Internet bookmarks, favorites folders, and emails, or mental such as a person who is considered by others to be an "encyclopedia" on various topics. Does that mean that individuals who are very knowledgeable are information hoarders? No, and they should not be classified as having a disorder. However, individuals who feel it is critical to read *every* piece of information that comes to them should consider speaking to a counselor.

In addition, gathering information for a decision is a key aspect of forming knowledgeable decisions. Taking the information learned and acting on it is much different than continuing to gather information with an inability to move forward. Looking at the previous example, it is a good idea to read about various therapists in your area if you are seeking a professional. Questions you may have include the level of education, the number of years of experience, certifications, and reviews from other clients. However, it is important to examine the data and make an informed decision in no more than a few days, rather than constantly digging for weeks or months.

? What does your friend or family member hoard? How many of these categories does he or she fall into?

Chapter 5: Types of Hoarding: An Overview

Conclusion

Hoarding is no longer limited to simply the "collection of stuff". It has become a disorder with impacts on numerous types of industries and individuals. The next section will look at "who" hoards.

Chapter 5: Types of Hoarding: An Overview

Notes

1. International OCD Foundation. (2010). *Types of hoarding*. Retrieved from http://www.ocfoundation.org/hoarding/types.aspx.
2. ASPCA. (2012). *Clark county Ohio—February 2011*. Retrieved from http://www.aspca.org/Fight-Animal-Cruelty/aspca-in-action/clark-county-ohio-february-2011
3. Hay, F. (2011). *Social: Forget digital coaching, Is digital syllogomania the next big thing?*. Retrieved from http://www.ecademy.com/node.php?id=162253.
4. Beck, M. (2012). Drowning in email, photos, files? Hoarding goes digital. *Wall Street Journal*. Retrieved from http://online.wsj.com/article/SB10001424052702303404704577305520318265602.html.
5. Samson, N. (2011). Bibliomania and the not-so-light side of book hoarding. *Quill and Quire*. Retrieved from http://www.quillandquire.com/blog/index.php/2011/03/31/bibliomania-and-the-not-so-light-side-of-book-hoarding/.
6. Reinardy, R. M. St Louis Obsessive Compulsive Disorder Support Group. (2006). Information hoarding: The need to know and remembering. *OCD Newsletter*. Retrieved from http://www.stlocd.org/handouts/InformationHoardingTheNeedtoKnowandRemember.pdf.
7. Beck, M. (2009). Super savers: Helping the hoarders. *Wall Street Journal*. Retrieved from http://online.wsj.com/article/SB10001424052748704500604574483480666149034.html.

Chapter 6: Who "Gets" OCD?

OCD is not a disorder that affects simply one group of individuals. It can afflict anyone. However, is it more prevalent in men or women? Is there a difference in the characteristics between children and adults? Is there an ethnicity, race, or socioeconomic barrier? This will now be discussed.

Prevalence refers to how common a disorder is, and in which demographics it is more likely to occur.

Socioeconomic status (SES) refers to an individual, or family's, income, education, profession, and residence.

Prevalence of OCD is lower than other anxiety disorders but is higher than what was previously assumed. Depending on the study, the prevalence rates of OCD vary from one to two percent of the population.[1] However, additional research is needed to continue to confirm these results. Also, these results may be biased as there are several individuals with OCD who do not seek treatment.

From the media examples provided earlier, it would be assumed that men are more likely to receive a diagnosis of OCD than women. Is that stereotype true?

Research on this area differs. Many studies have not shown any difference, with an equal ratio between males and females. However, one British study suggested that the ratio may be 1.4:1 with women being more likely to receive a diagnosis of OCD.[1]

Do children and adults differ in their display of OCD?

Research about children is slightly different than their adult counterparts. Due to the fact that this research is so important, especially to the parents of children who may be struggling with

Chapter 6: Who "Gets" OCD?

OCD, an entire chapter has been devoted to this area. See the chapter "A Special Look at Children" for more information.

What about other demographics including race, ethnicity, and SES?

A larger proportion of divorced, separated, and unemployed individuals appear to be diagnosed with OCD. However, this correlation may make more sense in reverse. OCD behaviors can cause serious strain in relationships and may make keeping a steady job difficult. Therefore, individuals diagnosed with OCD are more likely to fall into these categories.[1]

As you can see, the individuals suffering from OCD fit into several categories, not a specific stereotype. These differences are important to understand in order to grasp the various treatments available.

Notes

1. Bratiotis, C., Otte, S., Steketee, G., Muroff, J., & Frost, R. O. International OCD Foundation. (2009). Hoarding Fact Sheet. Retrieved from http://www.ocfoundation.org/uploadedFiles/Hoarding%20Fact%20Sheet.pdf?n=3557.

Chapter 7: Who Hoards?

Is there a group of individuals more likely to engage in hoarding behaviors? This chapter will look at the demographics of hoarders and a give brief overview of what may cause them to hoard. The prevalence of hoarding will also be discussed here.

Prevalence

Prevalence of compulsive hoarding varies from different studies. Some statistics quote two and five percent of the population may be suffering with severe hoarding problems.[1] Others report that 1.2 million people in the United States suffer from hoarding.[2] Another states that three million Americans are afflicted.[3] Further research states that only 700,000 to 1.4 million Americans are affected.[4] Unfortunately, it has proven difficult to locate legitimate research for countries other than the United States.

The population being studied also makes a difference. Between 18 and 40 percent of individuals seeking professional help for OCD may be compulsive hoarders, although they do not necessarily have OCD.[5]

Clearly, statistics vary drastically and much of this is dependent upon an individual's willingness to admit to needing assistance. However, it is clear that hoarding causes great anxiety to many people and their affects can carry over to loved ones, coworkers, and pets.

Age, Gender, and Other Demographics.

Research continues to show that the elderly are more likely to hoard, and the average age for an individual seeking treatment for these behaviors is 50.[1] However, hoarding may affect children, adolescents, and younger adults as well.[5] Some researchers believe the age of onset may appear during adolescence.[3] Others believe it may begin during childhood and adolescence but worsen during adulthood.[6]

33

Chapter 7: Who Hoards?

Some research studies have shown differences between genders in hoarders, whereas others have not. Usually, women are more likely to seek treatment for these behaviors than men, however.[5] It is difficult to know if women are generally more likely to hoard, or if they are simply more likely to believe they have a problem and to thus seek help.

Hoarders are more likely to live alone.[1] It is difficult to say if there is a direct correlation. Do those that live alone tend to hoard or do the hoarding practices cause that person to live alone? Research is still needed in this area and several others including gender, ethnicity, and socioeconomic status.

Categorization of Hoarders

The causes of hoarding will be discussed in depth later, but three "types" of hoarders have been proposed[7]:

1. The Indecisive Hoarder. This person does not find any decision can be made easily, and this includes the disposal of possessions.
2. The Frugal Hoarder. This person believes in the "waste-not-want-not" philosophy. She wants to keep everything so that she may turn it into something useful. However, this may never occur.
3. The Shortage Hoarder. This person worries that a disaster will occur that will impair the person's ability to buy necessary items such as food or household products. Therefore, he keeps anything he believes may be useful in the future.

❓ Which of these best describes the person that you know?

Conclusion

Research is still desperately needed in this area in order to thoroughly understand those that hoard. However, this disorder is

Chapter 7: Who Hoards?

getting more adequate attention and more information will hopefully be available in the near future. Next, we will take an in-depth look at OCD in order to better understand it and the individuals it affects.

Notes

1. Bratiotis, C., Otte, S., Steketee, G., Muroff, J., & Frost, R. O. International OCD Foundation. (2009). Hoarding Fact Sheet. Retrieved from http://www.ocfoundation.org/uploadedFiles/Hoarding%20Fact%20Sheet.pdf?n=3557.
2. University of California at San Diego. (n.d.). *What is compulsive hoarding*. Retrieved from http://psychiatry.ucsd.edu/OCD_hoarding.html.
3. The Compulsive Hoarding Center. (2012). *About compulsive hoarding*. Retrieved from http://www.compulsivehoardingcenter.com/Compulsive_Hoarding.html.
4. Borchard, T. (2012). 10 Things You Should Know About Compulsive Hoarding. *Psych Central*. Retrieved from http://psychcentral.com/lib/2011/10-things-you-should-know-about-compulsive-hoarding.
5. Mataix-Cols, D., Frost, R. O., Pertusa, A., Clark, L. A., Saxena, S., Leckman, J. F., ...Willhelm, S. (2010). Hoarding disorder: A new diagnosis for DSM-V?. *Depression and Anxiety* 27, 556-572.
6. Hartford Hospital. (n.d.). *Anxiety Disorders Center/Center for Cognitive Behavioral Therapy: Compulsive Hoarding*. Retrieved from http://www.harthosp.org/instituteofliving/anxietydisorderscenter/compulsivehoarding/default.aspx.
7. Chromy, B. J. (n.d.). *Compulsive hoarding* [PowerPoint Slides].

Chapter 8: OCD in Depth

Chapter 8: OCD: In Depth

Now that you understand some of the basics of obsessive-compulsive disorder, let's look at this disorder more closely. This chapter will discuss the suspected causes of OCD, the early warning signs that someone you know may exhibit, and the behaviors and symptoms associated with the disorder.

1) Causes

Research has now shown that causes for OCD can be biological, psychological, and even evolutionary based. First, biological causes will be examined including genetics, brain abnormalities, and neurotransmitter abnormalities. Next, a discussion of psychological causes including OCD behaviors that are learned, cognitive biases, and the attempt to suppress OCD obsessions will commence. Finally, we will discuss OCD and the benefits it has served from an evolutionary standpoint that are no longer necessary.

a) Genetics

There is now reason to believe that OCD may be, at least in some part, genetic. This was originally thought when numerous studies showed that family members of individuals diagnosed with OCD, also have been or could be diagnosed with the disorder. In fact, this number may be as high as 3 to 12 percent in immediate family members. Twin studies, which compare monozygotic (identical) to dizygotic (fraternal) twins, also show a strong correlation to indicate a genetic connection.[1]

Although there does not appear to be one specific gene related to OCD, certain genetic abnormalities do increase an individual's vulnerability to the disorder.[2] One of the genes, as tested in a study with mice, related to the compulsion to clean oneself, (such as hand washing,) is the gene SAPAPA3.[3] Additional research with humans is needed before this can truly be confirmed. This

Chapter 8: OCD in Depth

gene alone does not explain the obsessive thoughts associated with OCD, either.

It is important to understand that OCD, like most mental health disorders, is a product of both biological factors and environment. A person vulnerable to OCD may never actually show OCD symptoms.[2] Therefore, although genetic factors are important to understand so that scientists can adjust treatment methods, having a specific "OCD gene" is not a curse or something to fear.

b) Brain Abnormalities

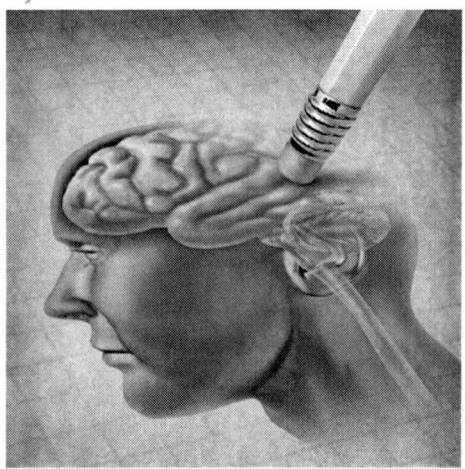

OCD, like many disorders, can be linked to abnormalities in the brain. As technology advances, our ability to explore the brain, and its abnormalities, grows.

Several parts of the brain have increased activity in individuals with OCD. This increased activity can cause specific compulsions, like those related to fear of contamination or fear of injury to others.[1]

c) Neurotransmitter Abnormalities

Similarly to brain abnormalities, there are those found in neurotransmitters.

Chapter 8: OCD in Depth

Neurotransmitters are areas of nerves that send signals to other nerves to transmit messages and follow-up actions. Neurotransmitters are intricately related to brain chemicals.

Serotonin and several other neurotransmitters have now shown a connection to OCD. An decrease in serotonin may result in OCD behaviors as well as depression.[1] Medication may help even out serotonin, but there may also be substantial costs, which will be discussed later.

Neurotransmitter abnormalities may not be enough by themselves to cause OCD. However, along with environmental influences and other genetic factors, they can have an effect.

d) OCD as a Learned Behavior

For lack of a better term, OCD "feeds" on itself. Individuals engage in compulsions because it decreases the anxiety they feel from their obsession. For example, a person who is distressed over a fear of germs will find a decrease in this stress after washing their hands. Therefore, the individual learns that engaging in these compulsions will soothe emotional distress. After learning this, the person will continue to engage in these behaviors, even if they are unhealthy, to decrease the stress. This may be one reason that it is often difficult to successfully treat OCD.[1]

e) Attempted Suppression of OCD

Some studies have attempted to help patients learn to suppress obsessions. This method has proven ineffective. When individuals are told to suppress these thought processes, they become even more obtrusive and distressing. Individuals may try to suppress these thoughts on their own in order to manage their anxiety, only to have the reverse effect.[1]

f) Cognitive Bias

Some individuals with OCD may struggle with blocking information and distractions that are not relevant. This inability to block may cause an attempt in emotional suppression, again,

Chapter 8: OCD in Depth

unsuccessfully. In addition, the individual may not feel confident in his ability to remember certain tasks, which adds to the need to repeat behaviors and check things.[1]

g) Evolution

Although it may seem strange now, OCD could have been extremely effective several hundreds of years ago. Due to the high rate in family members, scientists now believe that OCD may have ties to evolution.[1]

Grooming and hygiene acts that reduce stress may have once served a purpose of relieving stress during conflicts, as well as keeping clean.[1]

It would also make sense that during times when diseases were easily contracted from routine activities, individuals who paid close attention to remaining clean, would live longer, and therefore reproduce. At the time, these obsessions and compulsions may have been considered good hygiene and self-preservation acts, rather than a disorder.

2) Early Warning Signs

There are no true warning signs of OCD besides the symptoms of the disorder. That being said, the disorder's onset is most often gradual, steadily becoming worse with time. Therefore, any symptoms being exhibited are "signs" that the disorder is forming, and most likely progressing.

However, symptoms may increase and decrease over time. Therefore, the OCD may appear to be more severe at specific times and should be treated as such.

3) Symptoms and Behaviors

Symptoms and behaviors vary depending on which type of OCD the person has. In an earlier chapter, we briefly looked at the types of OCDs based on symptoms.[4] Let's explore each of those more closely now.

Chapter 8: OCD in Depth

a) Fear of Contamination (Cleaning)

Fear of contamination is generally the fear of germs on the self, others, or the environment.

An obsession regarding this fear may be a thought process involving the number of germs that could possibly be on the surroundings or believing that the person can feel the germs on their skin.

Compulsions associated with these obsessions may include:

- Bathing multiple times per day
- Requiring others to engage in certain cleaning and hygiene practices
- Cleaning the surroundings with a specific cleaner, with a certain technique, or a certain number of times.
- Washing hands repeatedly

? How often does the individual wash himself? Is it excessive? Is the house or apartment spotless beyond the standards of good housekeeping?

Simple fear of contamination is usually not associated with psychosis. If the individual experiences formication or a similar disorder, immediate medical attention should be sought. This is no longer a case of OCD.

Formication, also referred to as tactile hallucinations, is the feeling that insects are crawling on or under the skin, despite the fact that there is no physical evidence.

b) Checking

Constantly checking objects is another form of OCD with a specific behavior. That is that individuals will often "check" on things a certain number of times. For example, an individual may

Chapter 8: OCD in Depth

need to turn the stove on and off three times to feel confident that it is off.

This is especially common in relation to objects or circumstances that could be considered dangerous. For example, a stove that is left on could start a fire. A door left unlocked could invite intruders. A faucet left running could cause a flood in that room.

Therefore, this practice is entirely understandable. Many adults have been drifting to sleep and then walked to the door to make sure it was locked. They simply couldn't remember.

However, the difference between these two scenarios is the reason and practice of locking the door. See the following situations.

Sally: "Did I lock the door before lying down? Oh, I can't remember. I guess I should get up and check." Sally looks at the knob, sees that it is locked, and returns to bed.

Maggie: "Did I lock the door before lying down? I'm pretty sure I did. I think I did. Just in case, I better go check." Maggie looks at the knob, sees it is locked, and proceeds to unlock it and relock it three times. After engaging in this compulsion, she is able to return to bed.

It is obvious that Maggie has OCD while Sally does not.

The obsession is the nagging thought process regarding if the item was locked, turned off, etc. This thought process may continue, even though the individual knows that he has performed the action, until the action is repeated satisfactorily.

The compulsion is the behavior of constantly turning the knobs, pressing handles, and locking locks. Often, these behaviors must be performed a set number of times prior to the person feeling that the task is complete.

Chapter 8: OCD in Depth

❓ Does the person constantly have to check to make sure things are off, locked, or secure?

c) Counting

Counting is another common type of OCD and its symptom is exactly as it sounds: counting. Individuals may count the number of times they chew their food, the number of times they enter and exit a doorway, or the number of times they flip the light switch before leaving the room. This number may remain constant. (Linda must turn the stove off three times, the light switch off three times, and turn the key in the lock three times.) It may also slowly increase with time and what started as turning the knob twice has turned into turning it seventeen times.

This type of OCD can become dangerous if a person has to wait for a certain number of red and green lights before he can drive through an intersection. Although this may seem like an extreme example, it is not impossible, and can become life threatening.

❓ Does this person seem to count silently, or aloud, while he performs certain actions?

d) Ordering and Arranging

Ordering and arranging often come hand-in-hand. These practices may be with clothes hanging in the closet or with all the pencils having to be in an exact row. It may be that the dishes only belong in specific areas of specific cabinets, or that all the bedroom knick-knacks are arranged according to size on the bedroom dresser.

This does not mean that everyone who wants the plates in one cabinet and the glasses in another is OCD. This person is simply organized. However, there is a difference between organized and an OCD display of ordering. Later, we'll discuss the difference between normalcy and disorder.

Chapter 8: OCD in Depth

There was a teenager who refused to go to bed prior to setting his room "just the way I like it". His parents became frustrated as this child often had to stay up late. In frustration, they turned off the child's light at ten o'clock and he was not allowed to turn it back on. Instead of being able to lie down, the child worked in darkness or with the aid of a flashlight. He simply could not sleep, no matter how hard he tried, until everything was in order. Eventually, his parents allowed him to go to his room earlier to get his room ready before going to bed. This relieved stress in all parties.[1]

❓ When entering this person's house, room, or office, do the items appear to be "just so" all the time? Does he become upset when things are moved?

e) Repetitive Behaviors

Repetitive behaviors often go hand-in-hand with checking. However, this may extend past the checking procedures.

For example, a woman may feel she has to chew each bite of food twice on her left molars and twice on her right molars. Only being able to chew the food on one side or a limited or excessive number of times may prove to be overwhelming to her.

A man may feel that he needs to snap his fingers every time another person says the word "cake". This behavior may only be associated with this word and may not cause problems until a discussion regarding birthdays, weddings, or pastries is involved.

A child may feel that she needs to say the word "hello" three times upon greeting someone rather than once. Disturbance of this practice may cause her tremendous panic as she tries to continue the greeting.

The obsession is thinking that his behavior <u>must</u> occur due to a certain trigger. (The trigger could be a word, food, music, etc.) The individual feels that this action is mandatory.

Chapter 8: OCD in Depth

The compulsion is the individual engaging in the repetitive behavior, whether that is chewing the food correctly snapping, or restating words.

❓ Does the individual seem to engage in behaviors a set number of times or due to certain triggers?

f) Fear of Causing Harm to Others

An individual with OCD may have a horrifying fear of causing harm to others, especially those that he or she loves. This can be much more severe than simply believing that she will cause harm through physical means, but also due to superstitions.

This form goes along the old saying of "Step on a crack and break your mother's back", something that elementary children often say to one another. This can be followed by children trying to step anywhere on the sidewalk except for the crack.

To some children, this type of saying is a fun game. For children with OCD, they may have a dreadful fear of this actually becoming true. Therefore, they must try very hard to never step on a crack, regardless of the situation. Being pushed by another child that causes them to step on a crack may result in a tearful meltdown.

A man may feel that his wife will become ill, or die, if he does not turn the light switch on and off six times before leaving a room. He may logically know this to be false, but still feels compelled to protect her by performing the task anyway.

This is not the same as an individual believing that she will injure her spouse in her sleep due to being possessed or that she has no control over her left arm and therefore may punch people who get too close to her. This is a form of psychosis and appropriate medical attention should be sought immediately.

Chapter 8: OCD in Depth

Once a person has decided that the practice is somehow involved in the welfare of those around him, it may be incredibly difficult for him to stop the practice due to his fear that his family could die, be injured, or become ill. This particular form of OCD can be particularly difficult to treat.

The obsession is the constant fear of a loved one becoming injured or ill. Even despite knowing that low probability of this happening, the thought persists.

The compulsion is the person engaging in behaviors he feels are required including stepping on certain blocks, turning on and off the lights, or saying the same word upon entering a room.

In addition, a person may become so terrified of causing a traffic accident and injuring or killing a passenger or pedestrian that she stops driving. This decision can greatly impair a person's functioning, especially if she lives in an area that does not have public transportation. Although many drivers have a reasonable fear of causing harm to others, this fear is taken to the extreme in this particular case.

? Does this individual talk about the harm she feels will come to you or others if she does not do certain things?

g) Symmetry

Some individuals with OCD may become obsessed with symmetry. That is, they feel that all items must be even with others.

For example, a person may be obsessed with pencils forming a straight line where all of the erasers are at exactly the same point and the led at the same point, regardless of the number of pencils. This compulsion may require the person to sharpen pencils repeatedly until they line up correctly.

Chapter 8: OCD in Depth

Another example is an individual who will repeatedly erase what he has written because the letters were too tall, too short, too round, or unequal to the other letters.

In this case, the obsession is the thought process related to the order or exactness of the objects in the room. The person feels that the disarray must be corrected.

The compulsion is the action of lining up the pencils exactly or erasing letters. As the previous examples show, this compulsion can be extremely time consuming, as well as frustrating.

? Does this individual feel that things must be in a line, straight, or arranged equally to all other items?

h) Sexual Obsessions

Sexual obsessions are not the same as fantasies as they are not considered pleasant by the individual and often cause excessive anxiety and guilt. Often, these obsessions are related to the purely obsessive type of OCD discussed earlier. The individual will try desperately not to act on these obsessions.

Topics of these obsessions could be taboo subjects such as sexual acts with animals, violence, or even children. These thoughts are intrusive and unwanted which can result in severe stress, anxiety, and guilt.

In addition, people with this form of obsession may choose not to seek treatment for fear of being judged or ridiculed. They may also feel like there is no one in who they can confide. Therefore, obsessions such as this may lead to severe depression.

? Does this person ever talk about obsessions such as this? Does he seem preoccupied with an obsession that he is unwilling to discuss?

Chapter 8: OCD in Depth

i) Religious Obsessions

Religious obsessions are not to be confused with being devout. Individuals with these obsessions are so filled with anxiety that they do not receive any pleasure for participating in these compulsions.

Individuals may worry that they have offended God accidentally by saying the wrong thing, not participating in a religious activity correctly, or saying an incorrect prayer.

They may also worry that they have performed an immoral act, even if only small and by accident. Receiving too much change from a store clerk, and not catching the mistake until later, may translate to them as stealing.

The need to constantly be moral and please God can become an exhausting chore that increases anxiety immensely.

j) Rituals

Rituals have been discussed throughout this text. Rituals can include counting the number of times a light switch is turned on, or having all the clothes in the closet hung by type and color before going to bed.

However, rituals can also be mental. Mental rituals might include someone spending hours going over each detail of an event or conversation, or attempting to erase parts of the event that he or she does not want to remember. It can also include counting or list making without speaking aloud.

Many people have "morning" rituals such as: get out of bed, shower, drink coffee, dress, and go to work. However, to a person with OCD, a broken ritual can be extremely stressful and symbolize a breakdown in the rest of the day. If a person feels he must have one cup of coffee prior to getting ready for work and the coffee maker breaks, he may simply call in. He may stay home, filled with anxiety, or buy a new coffee maker, which may

Chapter 8: OCD in Depth

have to be identical to the broken one, so that it can fit in the exact same space.

Rituals can be time consuming and emotionally and psychologically exhausting.

k) Other Obsessions and Compulsions

Although this chapter has covered several types of obsessions and compulsions, there are numerous others that have not been discussed. This does not mean that they are not equally important or do not need treatment.

For example, a young child who is learning to read may become so distressed at missing a single word that he demands he start again at the beginning of the book, even if he was at the last page. This can cause just as much anxiety to the child and family members as many of the other types of OCD that have been discussed.

Now that OCD has been covered in depth, hoarding should be explained in the same way.

Chapter 8: OCD in Depth

Notes

1. Butcher, J.N., Mineka, S., & Hooley, J. M. (2010). *Abnormal psychology.* (14th ed.). Boston: Allyn & Bacon. pp. 206-216.

2. Kelly, O. (2010, August 23). *OCD and genetics: Genes are only a piece of the OCD puzzle.* Retrieved from http://ocd.about.com/od/causes/a/OCD_genes.htm.

3. Welsh, J. M., *et al.* (2007). Cortico-striatal synaptic defects and OCD-like behaviours in *SAPAP3*-mutant mice. *Nature* 448: 894-900.

4. OCD Types Website. (2011) *OCD Types.* Retrieved from http://www.ocdtypes.com/.

Chapter 9: Hoarding in Depth

Chapter 9: Hoarding In Depth

An overview of hoarding has already been given. In this chapter, the causes, early warning signs, and symptoms will be discussed more in depth.

1) Causes

Causes of hoarding can include environmental factors, biological abnormalities, or psychological errors. These causes will be discussed here.

a) Environment

Many individuals believe that severe poverty or previous hardship can result in hoarding. Research does not currently support this assumption.[1] However, research does support the notion that a traumatic event may lead a person to hoard. This event could be a flood that causes damage to possessions, a car accident, or childhood abuse. The traumas may not seem related, but friends and family members may notice a change in the handling of a person's possessions after the event.

b) Genetics

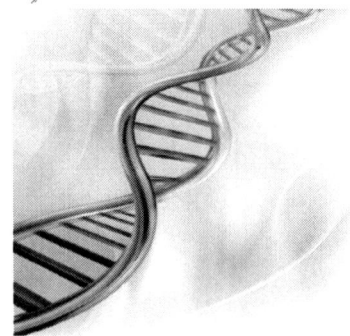

Some studies have proven that compulsive hoarding tends to run in families, making the case that there may be a genetic link in chromosome 14.[3,4]

Chapter 9: Hoarding in Depth

🔬In addition, one gene has been shown to correlate positively to both compulsive hoarding behaviors and to obesity. Additional research is needed to confirm these findings along with determining environmental factors that may contribute to both.[7] An additional gene was also linked with compulsive hoarding.[8]

🔬Hoarding and OCD have also been tested in rodents, in hopes of human focused applications. These studies have mixed results, which state that OCD, hoarding, and anxiety may or may not be genetic in rats.[9]

c) Brain Abnormalities
Some causes of hoarding may be biological, as brain imaging has shown that different areas of the brain have abnormalities between people with OCD and people with OCD with hoarding behaviors.[2]

d) Psychology
Some individuals hoard because they grow extreme emotional attachments to their possessions. This attachment may be more than to a single photograph, t-shirt, or memento. It could become an attachment to hundreds or thousands of possessions which results in the inability to discard anything.[5]

Others may hoard due to a perfectionist tendency. For example, they may be terrified of making mistakes in any decision and therefore refuse to make one.[5] If he believes that discarding the item is not entirely the right thing to do, he'll keep it. This thought process might be apparent in other areas in his life when asked to make a decision by friends, coworkers, or family members.

Hoarders may also be terrified that they will discard something of value and therefore will be unwilling to throw away anything.[5]

Chapter 9: Hoarding in Depth

For example, a cardboard toilet paper roll could be covered in peanut butter and rolled in bird seed so that it could be used as a bird feeder. Although the strange coin has no monetary value, a nephew might enjoy collecting coins. However, these plans will often never reach fruition and the house will remain cluttered with these objects.[5]

The inability to make a decision regarding possessions can be a symptom of trouble with information processing. Other signs of this include the inability to decide which possessions are valuable, and which are not, and difficulty remembering where things are. When hoarders have trouble remembering where they keep possessions, this may result in everything being kept in sight.[4] Therefore, things are left on the living room floor, rather than put on the top shelf of an empty closet.

A strong attachment to belongings is only one possible belief about the person's possessions. Additional beliefs may include the fear of forgetting about the possessions or the need to be in control of the possessions. Hoarders may become extremely distraught when another individual moves any of the belongings.[4] This can include discarding the possession, moving it to a different room or simply rearranging the furniture.

Hoarders can experience extreme emotional distress when faced with the possibility of discarding an item, or the inability to acquire an item they believe they want. In order to avoid this distress, they may refuse to make decisions about their possessions, including what to discard.[4]

? Which of these causes do you believe is the most likely cause of hoarding in the person you know? Was there a single event that

Chapter 9: Hoarding in Depth

seemed to trigger the behavior? Are other family members hoarders? Does there tend to be a problem with indecisiveness in other aspects of their life?

2) Early Warning Signs

Individuals may begin hoarding as early as childhood. Hoarders can hoard almost anything including practical possessions such as books, clothes, art, etc. or impractical things such as junk mail, plastic bags, or empty bottles. It is not uncommon for children or adolescents to have messy rooms and parents do not need to see a cluttered room as a sign of compulsive hoarding. However, if the child genuinely struggles with the inability to discard even the smallest and least significant of items, (such as candy wrappers, scraps of paper, bottle caps, etc.), a parent may want to consider seeking treatment.

As stated earlier, some people may hoard animals, which is characterized by having numerous animals without regard for genuinely caring for the needs of these animals, often to the point of neglect. If an individual begins to adopt or bring home a large number of animals but does not appear interested in caring for them, help for compulsive hoarding may be required.

In addition, if the collection of possessions begins to interfere with the person's functioning, it is time to research hoarding as a disorder, rather than simply a messy habit. See the chapter Crossing the Line: Normalcy versus Disorder for more information.

Chapter 9: Hoarding in Depth

3) Symptoms and Behaviors

Many symptoms and behaviors have already been discussed, so this section will serve only as a brief recap.

- The person may hold on to possessions once they are no longer useful.
- Animals may be collected in massive quantities, but then neglected.
- Individuals may become ashamed of their living arrangements and become socially isolated.
- Individuals may become severely distressed when faced with having to discard items, when items cannot be acquired, or when others move their belongings.
- Individuals may show extreme emotional attachments to possessions.
- Hoarding may impair a person's standard of living or quality of life.
- Hoarding may impair a person's health, including dangers in the house.
- A person may show signs of other disorders, including OCD.

? How many of these symptoms does the person you know exhibit?

a) Comorbidity

Hoarding has now been connected to dementia, especially in older adults. In addition, these individuals may suffer from anxiety disorders, such as OCD, mood disorders, major depression and substance abuse, as well as others.[5] These disorders will be discussed in the chapter of the comorbidity of hoarding. In

Chapter 9: Hoarding in Depth

addition to the dangers listed below, other dangers may be present when hoarding is combined with other disorders.

b) Dangers

Living in massive clutter may pose physical danger, especially to older adults who struggle with mobility. In some instances, this

clutter can result in falls that cause serious injury or death. Hygiene and health may also become a problem if individuals cannot access their refrigerators, sinks, stoves, bathtubs, or toilets. Although this may sound extreme, it is more common than originally thought.[3]

Social isolation, especially in older adults, may also be a concern.[3] Shame of the environment may cause individuals to not allow others in the house, which could cause them to slowly become isolated, often resulting in depression.

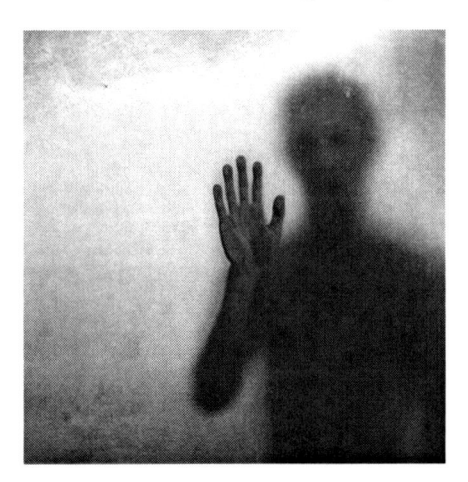

Seniors who hoard may face eviction due to these behaviors and be placed in a senior care center. This relocation could also be due

Chapter 9: Hoarding in Depth

to financial hardships from spending money on storage spaces or items that are hoarded. Some individuals also report difficulties in the workplace.[6]

Based on this information along with the brief overview, it is clear to see that hoarding can be a debilitating disorder that can cause hardships on numerous levels. Next, we will examine the factors in determining what constitutes a disorder.

Chapter 9: Hoarding in Depth

Notes

1. Bratiotis, C., Otte, S., Steketee, G., Muroff, J., & Frost, R. O. International OCD Foundation. (2009). Hoarding Fact Sheet. Retrieved from http://www.ocfoundation.org/uploadedFiles/Hoarding%20Fact%20Sheet.pdf?n=3557.

2. Butcher, J.N., Mineka, S., & Hooley, J. M. (2010). *Abnormal psychology.* (14th ed.). Boston: Allyn & Bacon. pp. 206-216.

3. Borchard, T. (2012). 10 Things You Should Know About Compulsive Hoarding. *Psych Central.* Retrieved from http://psychcentral.com/lib/2011/10-things-you-should-know-about-compulsive-hoarding.

4. Hartford Hospital. (n.d.). *Anxiety Disorders Center/Center for Cognitive Behavioral Therapy: Compulsive Hoarding.* Retrieved from http://www.harthosp.org/instituteofliving/anxietydisorderscenter/compulsivehoarding/default.aspx.

5. The Oprah Winfrey Show. (2005). Why Do People Hoard? Retrieved from http://www.oprah.com/home/What-Is-Compulsive-Hoarding.

6. International OCD Foundation. (2010). *Types of hoarding.* Retrieved from http://www.ocfoundation.org/hoarding/types.aspx.

7. Timpano, K. R., Schmidt, N. B., Wheaton, M. G., Wendland, J. R., and Murphy, D. L. (2011). Consideration of the BDNF gene in relationship to two phenotypes: Hoarding and obesity. *Journal of Abnormal Psychology. 120(3)*, 700-707.

Chapter 9: Hoarding in Depth

8. Alonso, P., Gratacòs, M., Menchón, J. M., Segàlas, C., Gonzálesz, J. R., Labad, J.,...and Estivill, X. (2008). Genetic susceptibility to obsessive-compulsive hoarding: The contribution of neurotrophic tyrosine kinase receptor type 3 gene. *Genes, Brain & Behavior. 7(7)*, 778-785.

9. Abramowitz, J. S., Taylor, S., McKay, D., and Deacon, B. J. (2011). Animal models of obsessive-compulsive disorder. *Biological Psychiatry. 69(9)*, e29-e30.

Chapter 10: Crossing the Line: Normalcy versus Disorder

Across this book, one theme is consistent: functionality. It is considered a normal act to check locks before going to bed, be a defensive driver, wash hands, and worry about the safety of loved ones. However, this becomes a serious problem when the obsessions or compulsions cause a person such distress that it impedes normal activity.

Here are questions a person may ask himself to assess if these habits have become a disorder:

- Do my cleaning rituals cause bodily harm such as washing my hands until they bleed?
- Do I have trouble sleeping due to intrusive thoughts? (This should be more common than simply occasionally worrying over a specific stressor such as a meeting at work the following day.)
- Must I check things such as locks, the stove, or light switches repeatedly prior to leaving the house or going to bed?
- Do I feel that my environment must be in a specific arrangement in order for me to sleep or continue my daily activities?
- Do I have specific routines that will cause me a great deal of anxiety to break?
- Do I hoard possessions to the point of filth or unnecessary disorganization?
- Do I realize that my behaviors or obsessions are unrealistic in nature?

Chapter 10: Crossing the Line: Normalcy versus Disorder

- Do I believe that my behaviors or obsessions are no longer under my control?
- Have my family members or friends commented on my behaviors being intrusive or obnoxious?
- Are my behaviors a burden to those around me?
- Have my behaviors caused me to become socially isolated?
- Are my obsessions or behaviors causing me anxiety or sadness?

Remember that research now shows that individuals with compulsions usually realize that these behaviors or thoughts are unrealistic, yet they feel that it is simply out of their control.[1] Others becoming angry and aggressive, which will only exacerbate, rather than alleviate, the problem.

If you feel that the behaviors or thought processes have reached the point of a disorder, it is time to consider seeking treatment.

Notes

1. Butcher, J.N., Mineka, S., & Hooley, J. M. (2010). *Abnormal psychology.* (14th ed.). Boston: Allyn & Bacon. pp. 206-216.

Chapter 11: What Other Disorders Are Common with OCD?

Certain disorders are more common in individuals diagnosed with OCD. This chapter will explain one mood disorder, four anxiety disorders, two personality disorders, and one somatoform disorder that are associated with OCD. Each of these disorders will be explained.

1) Major Depressive Disorder

The first disorder that will be discussed is major depressive disorder (MDD). Different sources report different findings ranging from one-third to two-thirds of individuals with OCD also suffering from MDD at some point in their lives.[1,2] In addition, depressive symptoms may occur in up to 80 percent of individuals diagnosed with OCD.[1]

What is MDD?

Symptoms of MDD include:

- An extended period of sadness
- A feeling of hopelessness
- Lack in interest in enjoyed activities
- Change in sleep patterns
- Change in eating behaviors

Chapter 11: What Other Disorders Are Common with OCD?

MDD can involve psychosis, self-injurious behavior, or suicidal thoughts or attempts. If any of these things occur, seek emergency medical assistance immediately.

How are MDD and OCD related?

The inability to control intrusive thoughts and compulsive behaviors can cause an individual to feel helpless and sad. These feelings can lead to MDD.

2) Anxiety Disorders

There are four anxiety disorders that are often comorbid with OCD: social phobia, panic disorder, generalized anxiety disorder (GAD), and posttraumatic stress disorder (PTSD). Each of these disorders has specific symptoms which affect people in different ways.

What is social phobia?

Social phobia is an intense fear of specific social situations such as public speaking, eating in public, or being surrounded by too many people.

In order to be diagnosed with this disorder, the person needs to feel panic or anxiety in these situations, often even when only thinking about them. The effects need to impair functioning in that individual as well.

Often, people with social phobias realize that their fear may be too extreme for the situation. This realization, however, does not diminish the anxiety.

How is social phobia related to OCD?

Chapter 11: What Other Disorders Are Common with OCD?

Individuals afraid of offending others, especially those with religious obsessions, may be terrified of social situations, including those in large groups.

What is a panic disorder?

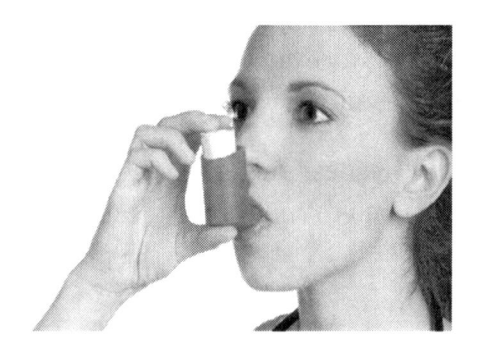

Panic disorder is a mental health disorder, in which panic attacks are frequent and seem to have no particular onset.

Panic disorder may be combined with agoraphobia, which is the fear of large crowds.

Panic attacks are characterized by a shortness of breath, sweating, choking, dizziness, and an overall feeling of fear.

How is panic disorder related to OCD?

People who have a fear of contamination, as more people are in one place, the more upset they will become, believing that excessive germs are present. In addition, becoming anxious regarding an obsession, especially if there is no outlet available for the compulsion, can result in a full panic attack.

Chapter 11: What Other Disorders Are Common with OCD?

What is GAD?

Generalized anxiety disorder is a mental health disorder in which a person *almost always* feels a sense of anxiety.

This may be characterized by someone who constantly worries about "the little things". Not only is she concerned with tomorrow's meeting, she worries about what she'll make for dinner, if the kids will get their homework done, if her husband will be late, is the dry cleaning done, etc.

People with GAD may be irritable, restless, and lose sleep due to this anxiety. They often find it difficult to control the levels of anxiety, as well.

How is GAD related to OCD?

Individuals with OCD may constantly feel anxious, especially if the OCD is severe. Constant list making, mentally deciphering events, or other rituals may be signs that this person is also experiencing GAD.

What is PTSD?

PTSD is an anxiety disorder that is more severe than acute stress disorder. PTSD is diagnosed after an individual has experienced a stressful and traumatic event that has had several devastating effects on the person's emotional, psychological, and physical wellbeing.

Acute stress disorder (ASD) is diagnosed during the first thirty days after the traumatic event. PTSD is diagnosed after the symptoms of ASD have persisted.

Chapter 11: What Other Disorders Are Common with OCD?

What symptoms are associated with PTSD?

Symptoms associated with PTSD include:

- Inability to concentrate
- Easily distracted
- Sleeping excessively or insomnia
- Hypervigilance
- Recurrent nightmares
- Flashbacks
- A constant state of fear
- Emotional numbness
- Irritability

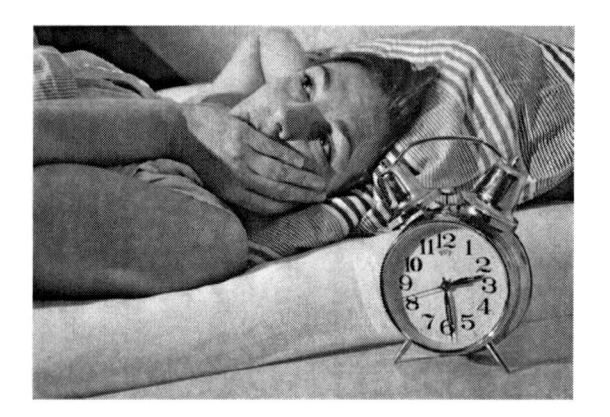

Hypervigilance is the state of being overly aware. This may include being easily startled, engaging in an overly vivid imagination, (usually against your control), or a need to check the environment for stimuli, (people or things,) associated with the traumatic event.

Chapter 11: What Other Disorders Are Common with OCD?

Flashbacks are similar to memories with one distinct difference: the individual feels that he or she is reliving the traumatic experience. During a flashback, the person may respond as if he is being traumatized including shaking, screaming, or even assaulting individuals around them. This is not intentional and often leads to high anxiety or sadness after the individual returns to reality.

How is PTSD related to OCD?

PTSD causes great anxiety in itself, and the OCD may seem secondary. However, the need to check things may build on itself. For example, a victim of domestic violence may feel she needs to check every room of the house, maybe even in some strange places such as the dishwasher or kitchen cabinets, to make sure the perpetrator is not in the building before she goes to bed. This can become a learned behavior and can eventually be a required part of her evening routine, even years after the abuse has occurred.[3]

3) Personality Disorders

What is dependent personality disorder (DPD)?

Dependent personality disorder is a mental health disorder characterized by a need to be taken care of due to feelings of being inept when alone.

People with DPD may avoid becoming angry, even when justified, with others due to a fear that the other person will leave them. This can lead them to remaining in an abusive relationship.

Chapter 11: What Other Disorders Are Common with OCD?

How are DPD and OCD related?

The anxiety associated with feeling that an individual may be abandoned, can cause certain compulsions and rituals including mental rituals of reviewing events.

What is avoidant personality disorder (APD)?

Avoidant personality disorder is a mental health disorder characterized by a fear of criticism that causes the person to avoid social situations, although they still desire affection and attention.

Individuals with APD may consider themselves socially inept and will go to great lengths to avoid social situations in which there is a possibility that they will not be liked. Even in intimate relationships, they may hold back important information to avoid being judged or shamed.

How are APD and OCD connected?

The anxiety of the two disorders may easily combine. People with OCD may purposely avoid situations that create anxiety, which can include social interactions.

4) Body Dysmorphic Disorder

What is body dysmorphic disorder (BDD)?

Body dysmorphic disorder is a mental health disorder in which a person is obsessed with his or her body, or a part of the body.

If an abnormality is present, the abnormality is grossly exaggerated. Often, no abnormality is present. The person may

Chapter 11: What Other Disorders Are Common with OCD?

spend hours inspecting him or herself and worries about what others think of this, real or imagined, abnormality.

How are BDD and OCD connected?

BDD may be a diagnosis applicable to as many as 12 percent of individuals diagnosed with OCD.[1] Individuals with BDD may engage in constant checking and ritualistic behavior in order to diminish the anxiety from their obsession. There is a possibility that biological causes underlie both disorders.[4]

? Does the person you believe may have OCD also exhibit any of the symptoms of other disorders listed above?

It is clear that this disorder can be combined with several other disorders, each with their own dangers. A chapter will be devoted to a brief overview of treatment options available if the affected individual has been diagnosed with multiple disorders.

Notes

1. Butcher, J.N., Mineka, S., & Hooley, J. M. (2010). *Abnormal psychology.* (14th ed.). Boston: Allyn & Bacon. pp. 206-216.

2. Kelly, O. (2010, August 23). *OCD and depression: Depression and OCD frequently occur with one another*. Retrieved from http://ocd.about.com/od/otheranxietydisorders/a/ocd_depression.htm.

3. Various observations and interviews.

4. Butcher, J.N., Mineka, S., & Hooley, J. M. (2010). *Abnormal psychology.* (14th ed.). Boston: Allyn & Bacon. pp. 284-287.

Chapter 12: What Other Disorders Are Common with Compulsive Hoarding?

Chapter 12: What Other Disorders Are Common with Compulsive Hoarding?

Some mental health disorders are common with compulsive hoarding. Some of these have already been discussed with the comorbidity with OCD, but will be discussed here again as their impact with hoarding may be different than with OCD. In addition, new disorders are introduced.

1) Mood Disorders

Just as major depressive disorder, (MDD) is common in patients with OCD, it is also common in people who hoard.[1] Another mood disorder that is common in hoarders is bipolar disorder (BPD).[1]

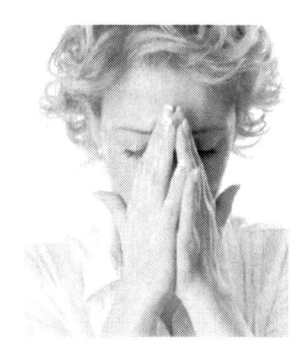

What is MDD?

Major depressive disorder is a form of depression that lasts several months, and is often present, at least in stages, through the lifespan

Chapter 12: What Other Disorders Are Common with Compulsive Hoarding?

Symptoms of MDD include:

- An extended period of sadness
- A feeling of hopelessness
- Lack in interest in enjoyed activities
- Change in sleeping patterns
- Change in eating behaviors

MDD can involve psychosis, self-injurious behavior, or suicidal thoughts or attempts. If any of these things occur, seek emergency medical assistance immediately.

How are MDD and Compulsive Hoarding related?

These disorders may be bidirectional. For example, a person who feels depressed and lonely, may begin to hoard or the person who hoards may feel depressed and lonely because of the behavior. Either of these can make the other worse and it may be a cycle that is only broken by treatment.

What is BPD?

Bipolar disorder is also referred to as manic-depressive disorder. That is, part of the time the patient is manic and at other points may be extremely depressed. During small windows, a person may seem "normal".

Symptoms of BPD include:

- A state of mania, which may last days or even weeks at a time
- A state of depression, which may last days or weeks at a time

Chapter 12: What Other Disorders Are Common with Compulsive Hoarding?

- A cyclic rotation of these states (Manic for two days, depressed for 18, and the cycle repeats)
- Possible psychosis, especially during mania
- A lack of sleep or appetite, especially during mania
- An inability to concentrate or stay still, especially during mania

Mania is a state of extreme hyperactivity in which a person may be unable to think or behave logically. Some individuals report being unable to experience pain, even if they hurt themselves while in this state, (such as burning themselves with cigarettes while smoking). Individuals in a manic state will often pace, ramble at high speeds, and become aggravated with others who try to calm them. In addition, they may experience visual or auditory hallucinations, perform self-injurious behaviors, break possessions, especially glass or mirrors, and spend large amounts of money on items that they do not need. They may feel that they do not need to eat or sleep and can function well without satisfying these physical needs. After the episode, individuals may, or may not, remember their actions in their entirety but confess that they did not feel like they could stop the behaviors from happening. It is not uncommon to have to hospitalize or sedate a manic person.

Hypomania is a state of lessened mania in which some symptoms are present, but are not yet severe. Hypomania is not discussed as much as mania or depression, because it is not always present in bipolar individuals. Many individuals suffering from BPD will switch from depressed to manic and vice versa without a transition phase. However, those that experience

Chapter 12: What Other Disorders Are Common with Compulsive Hoarding?

hypomania tend to believe it is the "best state" a person can be in. During this time, a person will require less sleep and food to be productive but will remain highly efficient without the possibility of psychosis, self-injurious behaviors, or spending excessive money. These individuals may only sleep from midnight to four a.m. and report feeling "refreshed" and ready to begin a day. They will then work on projects with great success. Other coworkers or their superiors may reward their high productivity, thus reinforcing this functional, yet unhealthy state. Although hypomania may remain for days or weeks, it is often a precursor to a full manic episode.

How are BPD and Compulsive Hoarding related?

First, a person may spend drastic amounts of money on possessions during a manic episode. For example, a bipolar woman once spent almost 1,000 dollars in a bookstore during a manic episode because "I had to have all of them right then" despite the fact that she knew she would never have time to read all of them.[2] If this habit is present and frequent, a person may accumulate a massive collection of items that were only impulse buys during the episode.

Second, during a state of depression, a person may hoard quite like a person diagnosed with MDD stated above. Their feelings of sadness or loneliness may be temporarily relieved with the purchase of new items.

2) Anxiety Disorders

There are two primary anxiety disorders associated with compulsive hoarding. The first is social anxiety and the second is posttraumatic stress disorder (PTSD).[1]

Chapter 12: What Other Disorders Are Common with Compulsive Hoarding?

What is Social Anxiety?

Social anxiety is a feeling of distress upon entering social situations. This distress may not be as intense as social phobia, (discussed earlier,) but is still alarming to the individual experiencing it. This anxiety may occur when the person must interact with a small group of coworkers, entertain others at his residence, attend a formal meeting, or grocery shopping.

Symptoms of social anxiety include:

- Emotional distress when surrounded by a small or large group of individuals, especially strangers
- Emotional distress when visualizing being in a social setting
- Physiological signs of distress including sweating, shaking, increased heart rate, or dry mouth

How are Social Anxiety and Compulsive Hoarding related?

Individuals who are terrified of social situations may feel more comfortable living alone amongst possessions. In addition, due to living alone, they may feel there is no need to keep the house orderly. Furthermore, they may not see that their compulsive hoarding is actually a problem, even if it interferes with their functioning.

What is PTSD?

PTSD is an anxiety disorder that is more severe than acute stress disorder. PTSD is diagnosed after an individual has experienced a stressful and traumatic event that has had several devastating

Chapter 12: What Other Disorders Are Common with Compulsive Hoarding?

effects on the person's emotional, psychological, and physical wellbeing.

Acute stress disorder (ASD) is diagnosed during the first thirty days after the traumatic event. PTSD is diagnosed after the symptoms of ASD have persisted.

Symptoms associated with PTSD include:

- Inability to concentrate
- Easily distracted
- Sleeping excessively or insomnia
- Hypervigilance
- Recurrent nightmares
- Flashbacks
- A constant state of fear
- Emotional numbness
- Irritability

Hypervigilance is the state of being overly aware. This may include being easily startled, engaging in an overly vivid imagination, (usually against your control), or a need to check the environment for stimuli, (people or things,) associated with the traumatic event.

Flashbacks are similar to memories with one distinct difference: the individual feels that he or she is reliving the traumatic experience. During a flashback, the person may respond as if they are being traumatized including shaking, screaming, or

Chapter 12: What Other Disorders Are Common with Compulsive Hoarding?

even assaulting other people. This is not intentional and often leads to high anxiety or sadness after the individual returns to reality.

How are PTSD and Compulsive Hoarding related?

As stated earlier, it has now been shown that traumatic events can trigger hoarding behaviors. These events may be abuse, neglect, a natural disaster, or vehicle accident. In addition, a traumatic event may worsen hoarding that was already present.

3) Dementia

As stated earlier, there has now been a connection drawn between dementia and compulsive hoarding, especially in older adults. Due to this fact, extra information will be given about this disease, including the various causes.

What is dementia?

Dementia is defined by a decrease in functioning, especially in memory and the ability to process information. The onset of dementia is gradual, but decrease in functioning is consistent and long-term.[3]

Symptoms of dementia include[3]:

- Memory loss
- Inability to recognize items
- Decreased motor functioning
- Difficulty organizing
- Difficulty planning

Chapter 12: What Other Disorders Are Common with Compulsive Hoarding?

What are the causes of dementia?

There are several disorders associated with dementia: Parkinson's disease, Huntington's disease, Alzheimer's disease, and vascular dementia. Other causes include stroke, brain injury, and being infected with HIV. More than 12 percent of dementia cases are reported to have more than one cause.[3]

Parkinson's disease occurs when there is a loss of dopamine neurons in specific parts of the brain. Upon this loss, the body will begin to have tremors and spontaneous movements. The prevalence of Parkinson's disease is higher in people over the age of 80, men, and nonsmokers. However, Parkinson's disease only occurs in one percent or less of individuals 60 to 69 and one to three percent of individuals over the age of 80. Dementia is likely to occur in 75 percent of patients with this disease. Parkinson's disease is believed to be the primary cause of dementia in 7.7 percent of cases.[3]

Huntington's disease is a disease that affects the central nervous system and results in spontaneous, involuntary motions that begin in one area of the body and then spread. The average age of onset is 40 and is equally common in men and women with a prevalence rate of approximately 1:10,000. Dementia is highly likely for people with Huntington's disease, which usually ends in death ten to twenty years after diagnosis. The cause of the disease is linked to chromosome four.[3]

Chapter 12: What Other Disorders Are Common with Compulsive Hoarding?

Alzheimer's disease is a neurological disorder that results in severe brain abnormalities. These abnormalities cause memory loss, impaired cognitive functioning, and deterioration of motor skills. It generally occurs after the age of 40 and the risk becomes higher with age, with approximately 30 percent of individuals over the age of 85 being diagnosed. Women are at a slightly higher risk than men to have the disease, which appears to be genetic. Alzheimer's disease will result in dementia and is eventually fatal. It accounts for more than 55 percent of all dementia cases.[3]

Vascular dementia presents symptoms similar to Alzheimer's disease but is due to blood being lost to specific areas of the brain for a short period of time. Age of onset is usually after the age of 50 and is more common in men. In individuals with dementia over the age of 65, vascular dementia may be the cause 19 percent of the time. Death may be caused by stroke or cardiovascular disease if medication is not prescribed.[3]

A stroke occurs when the brain does not receive enough blood, and therefore oxygen. This can be due to a blood clot in the brain or when an artery in the brain bursts. High blood pressure is associated with strokes. Strokes can impair motor skills, cognitive functioning, and memory. Strokes appear to be the primary cause in slightly less than 15 percent of individuals diagnosed with dementia.[3]

Chapter 12: What Other Disorders Are Common with Compulsive Hoarding?

Human Immunodeficiency Virus (HIV) is a blood condition, which drastically weakens the immune system and eventually leads to acquired immune deficiency syndrome (AIDS) and death. HIV can cause brain damage resulting in dementia. In addition, the body is more vulnerable to other diseases, which may also

cause dementia. Dementia can occur in more than 10 percent of HIV cases, with milder forms in up to 30 percent. In HIV patients, women are at a higher risk to develop dementia.[3]

How are dementia and compulsive hoarding related?

There are several other causes of dementia as well. From this brief overview, it is easy to see that dementia is likely to become a problem as an individual ages. Since compulsive hoarding tends to also increase, (or at least awareness of the disease tends to increase,) with age, it is not surprising that these two disorders would be correlated.

Individuals with dementia may forget what they've purchased, misplace items, be unable to organize, or want everything in the middle of the floor so that they can see it to remember it. All of these traits could lead to compulsive hoarding behaviors.

4) Attention Deficit Disorder
What is Attention Deficit Disorder?

Attention deficit disorder (ADD) is characterized by an inability to concentrate with thought processes quickly changing, which may result in memory problems. ADD can also have a hyperactivity component, which then becomes attention

Chapter 12: What Other Disorders Are Common with Compulsive Hoarding?

deficit/hyperactivity disorder, or ADHD, which includes an inability to stay still for an extended period of time.

Symptoms of ADD include:

- Inability to concentrate
- Changing thought processes, which may be considered as "daydreaming"

- An inability to remember specifics of conversations or events when attention was drifting, (not to be confused with short-term memory loss)

How are ADD and compulsive hoarding related?

At least one study has shown a correlation between ADHD in children with compulsive hoarding behaviors.[5] Another study showed a relationship between ADHD, PTSD, and compulsive hoarding behaviors.[6] However, PTSD may have some of the symptoms of ADHD including an inability to concentrate. Nonetheless, there does seem to be a relationship and additional research is needed to confirm these results.

5) Diogenes Syndrome
What is Diogenes syndrome?

Diogenes syndrome is characterized by severe self-neglect in the elderly.

Chapter 12: What Other Disorders Are Common with Compulsive Hoarding?

Symptoms of Diogenes syndrome include:

- Neglect of physical needs
- Apathy
- Social withdrawal
- Compulsive hoarding behaviors, often of trash

Individuals with this diagnosis are often intelligent and stubborn, which may result in refusal of treatment. The cause of this disorder is linked to stress, possibly to a single, traumatic event. [7]

How are Diogenes syndrome and compulsive hoarding related?

One of the key characteristics of Diogenes syndrome is the hoarding of trash. An unwillingness, or apparent cognitive inability, to discard of old newspapers, empty bottles, junk mail, etc. may be a sign of this disorder, as well as compulsive hoarding.

6) Other Disorders

Other disorders associated with compulsive hoarding include impulse control disorders and substance abuse. Impulsive eating and shopping may be associated with the tendency to hoard. In addition, approximately half of all compulsive hoarders have a history of abusing alcohol.[4] Additional research will be necessary to determine if this is purely a correlation, or also a causal factor.

? Does the person you believe may be a compulsive hoarder also exhibit any of the symptoms for other disorders listed above?

It is clear that this disorder can be combined with several other disorders, each with their own dangers. A chapter will be devoted to a brief overview of treatment options available if the affected individual has been diagnosed with multiple disorders.

Chapter 12: What Other Disorders Are Common with Compulsive Hoarding?

Notes

1. Hartford Hospital. (n.d.). *Anxiety Disorders Center/Center for Cognitive Behavioral Therapy: Compulsive Hoarding*. Retrieved from http://www.harthosp.org/instituteofliving/anxietydisorderscenter/compulsivehoarding/default.aspx.

2. Various interviews and observations.

3. Butcher, J.N., Mineka, S., & Hooley, J. M. (2010). *Abnormal psychology*. (14th ed.). Boston: Allyn & Bacon. pp. 206-216.

4. Mayo Clinic. (2011). *Hoarding Risk Factors*. Retrieved from http://www.mayoclinic.com/health/hoarding

5. Sheppard, B., Chavira, D., Azzam, A., Grados, M. A., Uma, P., Garrido, H., and Mathews, C. A. (2010). ADHD prevalence and association with hoarding behaviors in childhood-onset OCD. *Depression and Anxiety. 27(7),* 667-674.

6. Hartl, T. L., Duffany, S. R., Allen, G. J., Stekette, G., and Frost, R. O. (2005). Relationships amongst compulsive hoarding, trauma, and attention-deficit/hyperactivity disorder. *Behaviour Research and Therapy. 43(2)*, 269-276.

7. Reyes-Ortiz, C. (2001). Diogenes syndrome: The self-neglect elderly. *Comprehensive Therapy. 27(2)*, 117-121.

Chapter 13: What You Can Do if Someone You Know has OCD

Now that you have the necessary information about the disorder, you may wonder what you can do to help the person who you feel suffers from these disorders, or what the person can do to help themselves. Hopefully, this chapter will shed some light on your options as a friend or family member.

1) Who Can Diagnose It?

The first step to treating OCD is to have it diagnosed.

Although OCD can be diagnosed by a primary care physician, individuals that exhibit these traits are generally referred to a therapist or psychiatrist.

A therapist is a mental health professional who has received training in diagnosing and treating various disorders. Therapists can include psychologists, licensed clinical social workers, or an individual with a specific degree in counseling or marriage and family therapy. All therapists should have passed a licensing exam after completing a minimum of a bachelor's degree, although many also have masters and doctorate degrees. Ask for the qualifications of the therapist before beginning treatment.

A psychiatrist is a mental health professional who has received a medical degree (MD) and can prescribe psychiatric medication. This person attended medical school just as primary care physician, neurologist, or cardiologist. However, when this individual chose a specialty, he or she chose psychiatry and underwent specific training, including an internship and residency, in that field.

Chapter 13: What You Can Do if Someone you Know has OCD

§Although many insurance companies now understand the importance of mental health services, many still do not consider these services "medical". In addition, these plans may only cover a small number of sessions such as ten, twenty, or thirty per year. Insurance companies are more likely to cover psychiatrists since they have a medical degree.

§Not all therapists accept insurance and you may end up paying out-of-pocket. Look for a therapist with a sliding scale fee, which will help lower the cost for individuals with lower incomes.

§Expect to pay more for an initial visit, which may or may not be longer. Sliding scale therapists usually range from $40 to $80, with some charging much more. An initial visit may cost $140 to $170 or more.

§Talk to your accountant or tax preparer about taking a tax deduction for mental health services, which the United States government categorizes as medical expenses.

2) How is It Diagnosed?

The diagnostic and statistical manual (DSM) has undergone several revisions. The most current one is the DSM-IV-TR with the DSM-V expected to be released as early as this year. This book could be considered "the bible" of mental health disorders and is the primary text used to diagnose all disorders, including OCD.

The DSM gives very specific criteria for diagnosis, information regarding prevalence among age groups, genders, and other factors, and an overview of the disorder as a whole.

Therapists or psychiatrists will consult this text, although many know the symptoms of common disorders by heart, for the proper diagnosis and addressing the disorder accordingly.

Chapter 13: What You Can Do if Someone you Know has OCD

Insurance companies may insist on a diagnosis in order to establish payment.

Some individuals are hesitant to be diagnosed with a disorder, as they are worried that they will be "followed" by a "label". This is especially true of parents who worry about their children being stereotyped.

However, it is important that a person receives the correct diagnosis in order to receive the correct treatment. Some medications will exacerbate negative feelings if given to treat a different disorder. For example, medication for depression given to someone with bipolar disorder, may cause the person to become more depressed.[1]

In order to protect yourself or your child, pay close attention to the consent forms you sign. Often, there is one for your PCP in order for the therapist or psychiatrist to file for insurance. It is your choice if you release these records to anyone else including schools, employers, or family members. Therapy records are considered medical records and have special regulations even in a court of law. Discuss these concerns with your therapist if you feel they may be an issue.

3) What if Someone is in Denial?

Although many OCD individuals realize they have a problem, some still may not. If you feel that this person is in denial, it may be helpful to give an intervention.

Interventions are usually meetings in which a group of close friends or family members confront the individual directly and without warning. Often individuals take turns expressing how the person's behavior makes them feel. If the person realizes the negative effects he is causing to those around him, he may be more likely to enter some form of treatment.

Chapter 13: What You Can Do if Someone you Know has OCD

It is occasionally helpful to have a professional attend interventions. Although some therapists are willing to participate, there are professionals specifically trained in heading interventions. These professionals can be hired to assist you. However, they may be quite costly and do not expect insurance to pay for their services.

In preparing an intervention, it is important to have a structure and know what you will say beforehand. Many people find it helpful to write down their thoughts and read them aloud at the meeting. Be prepared for the confronted person to become angry or defensive, especially if the intervention happens without warning.

Undergo practices that you believe will best benefit the afflicted individual. Some people respond better when confronted with only one close friend, family member, spouse, or child, while others will be more apt to accept assistance if confronted by several people at once.

4) For Yourself

It is important to realize that dealing with a person—especially confronting a person—with OCD may be difficult on you as well. There are some resources available to you also.

First, you may want to consider individual therapy for yourself. Some people find that even a few sessions of talking to an empathetic professional gives them relief from the burden, especially if you are caretaker, and a sense of comfort.

You may also want to consider a support group. Check in your community to see if there are meetings available for family members or friends of people with OCD or other related disorders such as the disorders discussed in the previous chapter. If there are no groups available in your area, you may consider joining an

Chapter 13: What You Can Do if Someone you Know has OCD

online support group. Many people find that listening to people and sharing with others who are enduring similar struggles gives them a sense of unity, strength, and feeling of not being alone.

Seeking treatment is the first step in minimizing negative effects. It is vital to understand who can diagnose disorders, how they are diagnosed, and how to perform interventions.

Notes

1. Various observations and interviews.

Chapter 14: What You Can Do if Someone you Know Hoards

Chapter 14: What You Can Do if Someone You Know Hoards

Now that you have the necessary information about the disorder, you may wonder what you can do to help the person who you feel suffers from these disorders, or what the person can do to help themselves. Hopefully, this chapter will shed some light on your options as a friend or family member.

1) Who Can Diagnose It?

The first step to treating compulsive hoarding is to have it diagnosed.

Although you can discuss the situation with a primary care physician, individuals that exhibit these traits are generally referred to a therapist or psychiatrist.

A therapist is a mental health professional who has received training in diagnosing and treating various disorders. Therapists can include psychologists, licensed clinical social workers, or an individual with a specific degree in counseling or marriage and family therapy. All therapists should have passed a licensing exam after completing a minimum of a bachelor's degree, although many also have masters and doctorate degrees. Ask for the qualifications of the therapist before beginning treatment.

A psychiatrist is a mental health professional who has received a medical degree (MD) and can prescribe psychiatric medication. This person attended medical school just as primary care physician, neurologist, or cardiologist. However, when this individual chose a specialty, he or she chose psychiatry and

Chapter 14: What You Can Do if Someone you Know Hoards

underwent specific training, including an internship and residency, in that field.

§Although many insurance companies now understand the importance of mental health services, many still do not consider these services "medical". In addition, these plans may only cover a small number of sessions such as ten, twenty, or thirty per year. Insurance companies are more likely to cover psychiatrists since they have a medical degree.

§Not all therapists accept insurance and you may end up paying out-of-pocket. Look for a therapist with a sliding scale fee, which will help lower the cost for individuals with lower incomes.

§Expect to pay more for an initial visit, which may or may not be longer. Sliding scale therapists usually range from $40 to $80, with some charging much more. An initial visit may cost $140 to $170 or more.

§Talk to your accountant or tax preparer about taking a tax deduction for mental health services.

2) How is Compulsive Hoarding Diagnosed?

The diagnostic and statistical manual (DSM) has undergone several revisions. The most current one is the DSM-IV-TR with the DSM-V expected to be released as early as this year. This book could be considered "the bible" of mental health disorders and is the primary text used to diagnose all disorders.

Diagnostic criteria has been suggested for the DSM-V for compulsive hoarding to be classified as a separate disorder. These criteria include the collection of excessive items, an inability to discard items, and a decrease in functioning or quality of life. Specialists will also look for signs of dementia, Diogenes

Chapter 14: What You Can Do if Someone you Know Hoards

syndrome, and medical conditions to which the hoarding could be attributed.

The DSM gives very specific criteria for diagnosis, information regarding prevalence among age groups, genders, and other factors, and an overview of the disorder as a whole.

Therapists or psychiatrists will consult this text, although many know the symptoms of common disorders by heart, for the proper diagnosis and addressing the disorder accordingly.

$Insurance companies may insist on a diagnosis in order to establish payment.

Some individuals are hesitant to be diagnosed with a disorder as they are worried that they will be "followed" by a "label". This is especially true of parents who worry about their children being stereotyped.

However, it is important that a person receives the correct diagnosis in order to receive the correct treatment. Some medications will exacerbate negative feelings if given to the wrong people. For example, medication for depression given to someone with bipolar disorder, may cause the person to become more depressed.[1]

In order to protect yourself or your child, pay close attention to the consent forms you sign. Often, there is one for your PCP in order for the therapist or psychiatrist to file for insurance. It is your choice if you release these records to anyone else including schools, employers, or family members. Therapy records are considered medical records and have special regulations even in a court of law. Discuss these concerns with your therapist if you feel they may be an issue.

Chapter 14: What You Can Do if Someone you Know Hoards

3) What if Someone is in Denial?

Many individuals who hoard do not believe that they have a problem and will be resistant to advice and confrontation. If you feel that this person is in denial, it may be helpful to hold an intervention.

Interventions are usually meetings in which a group of close friends or family members confront the individual directly and without warning. Often, individuals take turns expressing how the person's behavior makes them feel. If the person realizes the negative effects he is causing to those around him, he may be more likely to enter some form of treatment.

It can be helpful to have a professional attend interventions. Although some therapists are willing to participate, there are professionals specifically trained in heading interventions, including those specializing in compulsive hoarding. These professionals can be hired to assist you. However, they may be quite costly and do not expect insurance to pay for their services.

In preparing an intervention, it is important to have a structure and to know what you will say beforehand. Many people find it helpful to write down their thoughts and read them aloud at the meeting. Be prepared for the confronted person to become angry or defensive, especially if the intervention happens without warning.

Undergo practices that you believe will best benefit the afflicted individual. Some people respond better when confronted with only one close friend, family member, spouse, or child, while others will be more apt to accept assistance if confronted by several people at once.

Professionals continue to advise that individuals speak in a calm voice and do not pass judgment on individuals who hoard. Express your concern without placing blame. Do not yell or insult

Chapter 14: What You Can Do if Someone you Know Hoards

the individual whom you are trying to help. It may be very helpful to discuss your strategy with a professional before the confrontation occurs.

4) For Yourself

It is important to realize that dealing with a person—especially confronting a person—with hoarding behaviors may be difficult for you as well. There are some resources available to you also.

First, you may want to consider individual therapy for yourself. Some people find that even a few sessions of talking to an empathetic professional gives them relief from the burden, especially if you are caretaker, and a sense of comfort.

You may also want to consider a support group. Check in your community to see if there are meetings available for family members or friends of people with compulsive hoarding or other related disorders such as the disorders discussed in the previous chapters. If there are no groups available in your area, you may consider joining an online support group. Many people find that listening to people and sharing with others who are enduring similar struggles gives them a sense of unity, strength, and feeling of not being alone.

Seeking treatment is the first step in minimizing negative effects. It is vital to understand who can diagnose disorders, how they are diagnosed, and how to perform interventions.

Notes

1. Various observations and interviews.

Chapter 15: Treatments for OCD

Treatments, like types and symptoms, vary greatly and each can be beneficial if used in the right context. It's important to remember that treatments are not a one-size-fits-all and a person may need to be patient while different treatments are attempted.

So what are the different types of treatment? Medication, psychotherapy, lifestyle changes, alternative medicine, and surgery will all be discussed in this chapter. In addition, benefits and risks will be discussed throughout.

1) Medication

Some medications known as selective serotonin reuptake inhibitors (SSRIs) may provide relief from OCD symptoms by regulating the amount of serotonin the brain produces. SSRIs are common in anti-depressant medication and can treat OCD and depression simultaneously.

Disadvantages of this medication include:

- Possibly up to half of clients will not feel significantly better.
- Once taken off the medication, between 50 and 90 percent of patients may return to previous symptoms.
- Although some studies have shown that medication and therapy combined help children,[2] other studies state that adults may have the same treatment outcomes from therapy only without medication.[1]
- Research is still being conducted regarding medication and hoarding behavior. At this time it appears that medication may reduce symptoms of comorbid illnesses, such as depression, but will not eliminate hoarding behaviors themselves.[5,6]

Chapter 15: Treatments for OCD

2) Psychotherapy

Behavioral and cognitive-behavioral therapy approaches have both been found to be highly effective. Often, clients are asked to confront their fears, such as touching dirty areas, such as the bottom of their shoes, and then not washing their hands.

Although many people may refuse this treatment, it has proven highly effective with reduction in symptoms in up to 75 percent of patients with the majority continuing to have success several years after treatment.[1]

Although this type of treatment may seem upsetting to some, the success rates are generally worth the risks.

3) Lifestyle Changes

Some individuals have found that lifestyle changes make living with OCD easier. Some of these changes include:

- Learning tools, (often in therapy,) to minimize compulsions
- Finding alternative methods. For example, an individual may attempt to realize that mowing the lawn can be just as effective, and far less time consuming, than trying to have all the blades match in height by cutting it by hand.
- Exercising may cause an elevated mood which may help individuals continue through the day with less anxiety.[3]

Chapter 15: Treatments for OCD

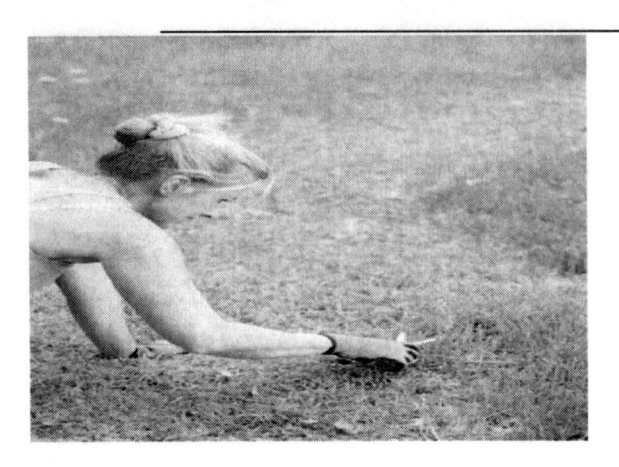

4) Alternative Medicine

In addition to medication, certain herbs, such as passiflora, may help to balance serotonin levels, causing relief from some OCD symptoms.[4] Also, some believe that OCD is caused by an imbalance in various organs and that the consumption of specific herbs can minimize these symptoms.[7]

In addition, yoga has found to help relieve obsessive thoughts, at least temporarily, with some poses working better than others.[4]

Furthermore, acupuncture may help relieve OCD symptoms when the pressure is applied to the areas of the liver, stomach, and spleen.[4]

5) Surgery

Surgery is not recommended for OCD except in severe cases, where OCD has caused extreme, negative effects and other treatment has been repeatedly unsuccessful. However, this criteria may fit up to 10 percent of OCD cases. In neurosurgery, a part of the brain that controls some of the OCD behaviors is deadened. The success rate for surgery reducing symptoms by at least one-third is about 35 to 45 percent.[1]

Some of these treatments may also assist individuals with compulsive hoarding, as the next chapter will discuss.

Chapter 15: Treatments for OCD

Notes

1. Butcher, J.N., Mineka, S., & Hooley, J. M. (2010). *Abnormal psychology.* (14th ed.). Boston: Allyn & Bacon. pp. 206-216.

2. Mash, E. J. & Wolfe, D. A. (2010). Abnormal child psychology. (4th ed.) Belmont, CA: Wadsworth. pp. 206-209.

3. Various observations and interviews.

4. Walding, A. Lance Armstrong Foundation. (2010, May 5). *Alternative treatments for OCD.* Retrieved from http://www.livestrong.com/article/117098-alternative-treatments-ocd/.

5. Bratiotis, C., Otte, S., Steketee, G., Muroff, J., & Frost, R. O. International OCD Foundation. (2009). Hoarding Fact Sheet. Retrieved from http://www.ocfoundation.org/uploadedFiles/Hoarding%20Fact%20Sheet.pdf?n=3557.

6. International OCD Foundation. (2010). *Types of hoarding.* Retrieved from http://www.ocfoundation.org/hoarding/types.aspx.

7. Browne, C. *Chinese herbs for OCD: Obsessive compulsive disorder in Chinese medicine.* Retrieved from http://www.agelessherbs.com/chineseherbsfor/ocd.html.

Chapter 16: Treatments for Compulsive Hoarding

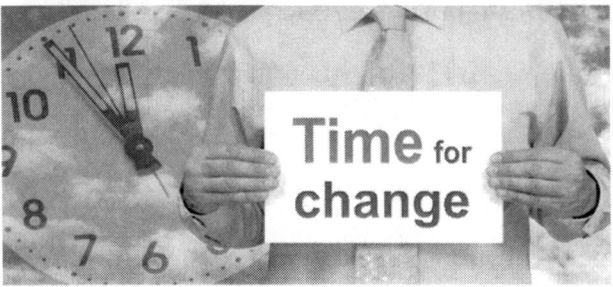

Just as there are several treatments for OCD, there are also a plethora of treatments for compulsive hoarding. This chapter will discuss medication, psychotherapy, lifestyle changes, and alternative medicine.

1) Medication

If the cause of hoarding is biological, such as an imbalance of brain chemicals, medications may prove very effective. Studies testing the effects of selective serotonin uptake inhibitors (SSRIs) have had mixed results.[1] It is also difficult to know if these medications work better on hoarders with OCD, rather than as a separate disorder. Additional research is required in this field.

In addition, SSRIs may cause dependence and can have negative side effects including depression and suicidal thoughts. Even if medication is used, additional treatment is mostly likely required.

2) Psychotherapy

Therapeutic interventions for compulsive hoarding have proven effective, although the techniques used will vary. These include traditional psychotherapy, such as cognitive-behavioral therapy, hands-on interventions inside the individual's home (supervised

Chapter 16: Treatments for Compulsive Hoarding

by a professional organization or therapist) group therapy, and family therapy.

Traditional psychotherapy, such as the use of cognitive-behavioral therapy in individual sessions, can help an individual understand errors in thinking processes. The client may also discuss other stressful conditions or traumatic events that may be linked to the hoarding behaviors.

Hands-on intervention is often required with compulsive hoarding cases. Therapists may visit the client's residence and help them organize their possessions while discarding irrelevant items. Many sessions may be required, especially in extreme cases. In addition, professional organizers can be hired to assist individuals with compulsive hoarding to clean their houses.

Family therapy may be helpful in order for members to understand the effects of compulsive hoarding on one another, especially those that co-reside. Therapists may be able to provide tools to help all family members live with less tension.

Group therapy can provide support and new ideas to struggling individuals. This may be especially true in groups that have members who have already overcome hoarding behaviors and feel the benefits of this change.

Clients who are forced into therapy, and therefore are not willing participants, may make very little or no progress. A mental health professional may become frustrated if they believe that the client has no motivation to change. It is important that clients are able to identify the problem, prior to seeking treatment.

Chapter 16: Treatments for Compulsive Hoarding

3) Lifestyle Changes

Some lifestyle changes can be highly effective in managing hoarding behaviors. These include:

- Finding an effective organizational system
- Setting a budget for spending on nonessential items

Finding an effective organizational system may prove especially difficult in the beginning. The first step is to discard any trash and clear enough space to be able to decide on places for useful kept items. For example, important mail may be placed on the left dining room table, but this is a moot point if it is still covered in other possessions.

Financial crisis is often a factor for individuals who spend excessive amounts of money on unused items. For example, a person suffering from bibliomania may spend hundreds of dollars on books each month. It is important for an individual to be able to see all of his necessary expenses, (e.g. food, housing, utilities, insurance, etc.) in order to see the amount of money remaining for extraneous items. This visualization will allow the person to see how much money would be available to be spent on items such as eating out, vacations, or a new computer, if money was not spent on books or other hoarded items.

4) Alternative Medicine

Some believe that the hoarding of items occur when there is an imbalance in the heart and that herbal supplements may assist in decreasing the hoarding tendencies.[2]

If anxiety is a root cause of hoarding, relaxation techniques may assist in minimizing the anxiety, and thus hoarding behaviors.

Chapter 16: Treatments for Compulsive Hoarding

These techniques may include breathing exercises, meditation, or yoga.

Overall, hoarding is difficult to treat until the individual believes that there is a problem and is willing to accept help. Others should <u>never</u> discard the person's items without his consent and this can cause extensive anxiety and anger. It is key that the afflicted person be an active participant in their treatment.

In addition to treating OCD and compulsive hoarding, it may also be beneficial to treat comorbid disorders. The next chapter looks at this extensively. Notes

1. Science Daily. (Oct 25, 2006). SRI medication effective in treating compulsive hoarding patients. Retrieved from http://www.sciencedaily.com/releases/2006/10/061024214706.htm.

2. Browne, C. *Chinese herbs for OCD: Obsessive compulsive disorder in Chinese medicine.* Retrieved from http://www.agelessherbs.com/chineseherbsforocd.html.

Chapter 17: Treatments for Associated Disorders

A lot of other disorders have been discussed in this book. It is common for an individual to be diagnosed with multiple disorders, and the treatments for these disorders could be different. For example, if a person had a phobia of snakes, showing them pictures of cows would most likely prove less than helpful, unless the person was scared of snakes *and* cows.

This chapter will give a brief overview of treatments for various mood disorders, anxiety disorders, personality disorders, and others listed in previous chapters. Positive and negative effects of each treatment type will also be discussed. However, this is not medical advice and any medications used should be discussed with a medical professional. In addition, prescription medications, non-prescription medications, and herbal supplements can have a negative and occasionally fatal combination. Let a doctor or psychiatrist know of any medications you may be taking or have previously taken.

1) Major Depressive Disorder

The first well-known treatment for MDD is antidepressant medications. These have gotten both popular in use and criticism in recent years, (for example the book *The Prozac Nation*). However, many primary care physicians and psychiatrists prescribe antidepressants, especially selective serotonin reuptake inhibitors (SSRIs), which increase the level of serotonin in the brain, which is often lower in depressed individuals.

Positive: SSRIs do increase hormones in the brain that should elevate the person's mood. This can have positive effects for many people, both in short and long-term cases.

Chapter 17: Treatments for Associated Disorders

Negative: There is often concern when prescribing antidepressants to children and adolescents, as the medication may make the patient more depressed, or even suicidal. Dependence on these medications can occur if they are prescribed for an extended period of time, often years. In addition, the medication may have minimal or no effect if not combined with psychotherapy.

The second treatment for MDD is psychotherapy. This treatment can occur in an individual, family, or group setting. The client generally visits a therapist or psychiatrist for the sessions. Cognitive-behavioral therapy is one type of psychotherapy used.

Positive: Psychotherapy can help a patient view the events or stressors differently. This can lead to relief of the pain simply from talking to a trained professional. Family therapy can help each member feel more empathetic towards one another and be able to develop positive relationship skills. Group therapy may help a person feel less alone and more supported. Assistance with admission to a psychiatric hospital can also be a helpful, positive quality from a professional who is aware of the patient's case.

Negative: Individuals who are skeptical of professional treatment may not find the method helpful. Some individuals may need medication in addition to the treatment due to biological abnormalities. Ill-trained therapists may not provide the necessary tools to help the patient help him or herself.

The third treatment option is electroconvulsive therapy. This is an extreme form of treatment in which volts of electricity are sent through the brain while the individual is sedated. This is usually only used for individuals who are suicidal, refusing to eat, or refusing to drink.[1]

Chapter 17: Treatments for Associated Disorders

Positive: This method can be helpful for a short period of time in extreme cases.

Negative: Success rates with this method are very low.[2] Additional treatment is highly recommended including medication and psychotherapy.

The fourth treatment alternative is inpatient hospitalization. Hospitalization can be either acute (generally four to 14 days), or long-term, (generally at least four months).

Positive: Hospitalization can provide a safe environment for patients to receive medication management, (especially if miss-medication has resulted in a severe depressive episode), and individual and group therapy. Trained professionals are immediately available for suicidal thoughts or attempts, aggressive outbursts, or other physical or emotional symptoms. In addition, family members may feel relieved that professional assistance is available and they do not have to try to keep the person safe.

Negative: Inpatient treatment is often very costly and insurance companies will pay very little of the bill, if any. In addition, adult treatment is usually voluntary and patients will not be admitted without consent and the ability to be discharged if they change their mind. This can be prevented by a court order, which is difficult to ascertain most of the time unless the person is declared insane, which can be a devastating opinion and "follow" the person on paper.

Note: If you honestly believe an individual may need professional help during an episode, call the person's current therapist. Most therapists will give an on-call emergency number. If you cannot

Chapter 17: Treatments for Associated Disorders

reach the professional or feel that the person is in immediate danger to himself or those around him, call the emergency services. An ambulance can be notified to transport the individual to a local medical hospital, which should have a psychiatrist or other mental health professional available to assess the patient and decide if additional mental health hospitalization is necessary. Intake to a psychiatric hospital can take a couple of hours and you may be required to sign forms admitting the patient, including those that state you are financially responsible for the stay. Carefully read anything you sign and discuss financial responsibility with hospital staff if it becomes an issue.

The last treatment possibility is routine exercise. This can include light walking, jogging, swimming, or use of fitness equipment.

Positive: Exercise naturally increases hormones that elevate mood. The brain may see this as a "natural high" and respond favorably.

Negative: Motivation for exercise can be a problem, especially if not participated in previously. In addition, individuals with previous injurious or chronic pain, such as from fibromyalgia, or muscular atrophy, may find exercise difficult.

2) Bipolar Disorder

The primary group of medications used to treat bipolar disorder is that of mood stabilizers. The original medication found to treat bipolar disorder was Lithium which showed usefulness in calming manic episodes and prevention of additional incidents.[3,4] The most recent medication that is receiving research regarding effectiveness in controlling BPD, especially in patients with depression, is Lamictal.[5,6]

Chapter 17: Treatments for Associated Disorders

Positive: Some medications have proven extremely effective in leveling bipolar episodes. Stabilization of brain chemicals may be required in some individuals, especially since BPD is often a lifelong condition. Newer medications are now considered to be safer than some of the "old-school" medications.

Negative: Some of the older medications may have negative health effects if used for an extended period of time for certain patients. Finding the correct dosage may be difficult in the beginning and require several weeks and visits to correct. Medications can have reverse effects including increase in depression and suicidal ideations. Many bipolar individuals do not like being on medication, as they prefer the "high" of mania or hypomania. Therefore, some patients may not be compliant with medication.

The second treatment option is psychotherapy. Again, this may be in the form of individual, family, or group therapy with a qualified specialist. Cognitive-behavioral therapy is often used.

Positive: Some individuals find that discussing their current life issues can be very cathartic. Family therapy may help each member empathize with the other and build tools for future episodes or daily living. Support groups may help the individual relate to others who experience the same disorder. It is most helpful if the therapist or psychiatrist can be reached via phone if the individual enters a severe manic or depressed episode. Assistance with admission to a psychiatric hospital can also be a helpful, positive quality from a professional who is aware of the patient's case.

Negative: Individuals skeptical about therapy may find the treatment very unsatisfying. Patients may be highly difficult to

Chapter 17: Treatments for Associated Disorders

calm during a manic episode, especially via phone but often also in person, even by a professional. Due to the chronic state of BPD, psychotherapy may take several years, at least on an intermittent basis.

The third treatment option is inpatient hospitalization. Hospitalization can be either acute (generally four to 14 days), or long-term, (generally at least four months). Acute hospitalization is especially common with severe manic episodes in which a person may be unable to calm themselves down without strong medication.

Positive: Hospitalization can provide a safe environment for patients to receive medication management, (especially if miss-medication has resulted in a severe manic or depressive episode), and individual and group therapy. Trained professionals are immediately available for suicidal thoughts or attempts, aggressive outbursts, or other physical or emotional symptoms. In addition, family members may feel relieved that professional assistance is available and they do not have to try to keep the person safe.

Negative: Inpatient treatment is often very costly and insurance companies will pay very little of the bill, if any. In addition, adult treatment is usually voluntary and patients will not be admitted unless they give consent and can be discharged if they change their mind. This can be prevented by a court order, which is difficult to ascertain most of the time unless the person is declared insane, which can be a devastating opinion and "follow" the person on paper.

Note: If you honestly believe an individual may need professional help during an episode, call the person's current therapist. Most

Chapter 17: Treatments for Associated Disorders

therapists will give an on-call emergency number. If you cannot reach the professional or feel that the person is in immediate danger to himself or those around him, call the emergency services. An ambulance can be notified to transport the individual to a local medical hospital, which should have a psychiatrist or other mental health professional available to assess the patient and decide if additional mental health hospitalization is necessary. Intake to a psychiatric hospital can take a couple of hours and you may be required to sign forms admitting the patient, including those that state you are financially responsible for the stay. Carefully read anything you sign and discuss financial responsibility with hospital staff if it becomes an issue.

The last treatment option is a change in lifestyle habits including a change in diet and exercise. Some professionals may recommend reducing caffeine or sugary foods, especially when a manic stage is expected.

Positive: The reduction of sugar and caffeine may result bursts of energy caused by these foods. Exercise can increase hormones that can naturally elevate an individual's mood during a mild to moderate depressive episode.

Negative: Motivation may be difficult for many people. This is especially true if the individual has a physical disorder that makes exercising painful.

3) Social Anxiety and Social Phobia

The primary group of medications used to treat social anxiety is that of SSRIs. These are the same medications used to treat depression and may have strong effects in reducing anxiety. Benzodiazepines may also be used in some chronic cases.

Chapter 17: Treatments for Associated Disorders

Different medications and/or dosages may be used for patients with mild social anxiety versus severe social phobia.

Positive: SSRIs may decrease anxiety while increasing or leveling mood. Individuals with chronic anxiety may find these highly effective.

Negative: Some of the older medications, especially benzodiazepines, may have negative health effects if used for an extended period of time on certain patients; including dependence.[7] Medications can have negative side effects, depending on the drug.

The second treatment option is psychotherapy. Again, this may be in the form of individual, family, or group therapy with a qualified specialist. Cognitive-behavioral therapy is often used.

Positive: Some individuals find that discussing their current life issues can greatly reduce their anxiety. Therapists may also assist individuals in facing specific social phobias such as large crowds or public speaking. Family therapy may help each member empathize with the other. Support groups may help the individual relate to others who experience the same disorder. It is most helpful if the therapist or psychiatrist can be reached via phone if the individual enters a severe episode such as feeling "trapped" at a supermarket. It may be helpful for a patient to carry the therapist's contact number and instructions in their wallet to call them. As a result, during an episode, another individual, such as a paramedic, may be able to locate the therapist for additional assistance.

Chapter 17: Treatments for Associated Disorders

Negative: Individuals skeptical about therapy may find the treatment very unsatisfying. It may take several sessions for an individual to be able to calm his anxiety.

The last treatment option is the act of meditation, relaxation, yoga, or breathing exercises.

Positive: Relaxation exercises can help to naturally calm anxiety, especially when a panic attack may be anticipated. An individual may also feel that beginning the day with these rituals could help in staying calmer during daily tasks including working, shopping, and attending events.

Negative: Individuals skeptic of these practices may find them less than useful. It may take time to learn various techniques, which may not provide immediate assistance.

4) Panic Disorder

The primary group of medications used to treat panic disorder is that of SSRIs. These are the same medications used to treat depression, and other anxiety disorders, and may have strong effects in reducing anxiety. Benzodiazepines may also be used in some chronic cases.

Positive: SSRIs may decrease anxiety while increasing or leveling mood. Individuals with chronic anxiety may find these highly effective. Benzodiazepines have a fast onset and may reduce a panic attack more quickly.

Negative: Some of the older medications, especially benzodiazepines, may have negative health effects if used for an extended period of time in certain patients; including dependence.

Chapter 17: Treatments for Associated Disorders

Medications can have negative side effects, depending on the drug.

The second treatment option is psychotherapy. Again, this may be in the form of individual, family, or group therapy with a qualified specialist. Cognitive-behavioral therapy is often used.[8,9] In addition, assisting a client to act out the symptoms of a panic attack can be used.[10]

Positive: Some individuals find that discussing their current life issues can greatly reduce their anxiety. Therapists may also assist individuals in facing specific phobias such as fear of heights, spiders, or closed spaces. Family therapy may help each member empathize with the other and create a safety plan for panic attacks. Support groups may help the individual relate to others who experience the same disorder. It is most helpful if the therapist or psychiatrist can be reached via phone if the individual enters a severe episode such as feeling "trapped" when faced with a specific fear. It may be helpful for a patient to carry the therapist's number and instructions in their wallet to call if needed. As a result, during an episode, another individual, such as a paramedic, may be able to locate the therapist for additional assistance. Practicing the common states of a panic attack may relieve anxiety during future attacks.[10]

Negative: Individuals skeptical about therapy may find the treatment very unsatisfying. It may take several sessions for an individual to be able to calm his anxiety. Many clients may decline therapy when forced to face their fears directly, such as holding a spider.

The last treatment option is the act of meditation, relaxation, yoga, or breathing exercises.

Chapter 17: Treatments for Associated Disorders

Positive: Relaxation exercises can help naturally calm anxiety, especially immediately before or during a panic attack. An individual may also feel that beginning the day with these rituals could help in staying calmer during daily tasks including working, shopping, and attending events. Individuals may also use these techniques before sleeping in order to sleep well.

Negative: Individuals skeptic of these practices may find them less than useful. It may take time to learn various techniques, which may not provide immediate assistance.

5) Generalized Anxiety Disorder

The primary group of medications used to treat GAD is that of SSRIs, although other drugs may also be taken. These are the same medications used to treat depression, and other anxiety disorders, and may have strong effects in reducing anxiety. Benzodiazepines may also be used in some chronic cases.

Positive: SSRIs may decrease anxiety while increasing or leveling mood. Individuals with chronic anxiety may find these highly effective.

Negative: Some of the older medications, especially benzodiazepines, may have negative health effects if used for an extended period of time in certain patients; including dependence.[11] Medications can have negative side effects, depending on the drug.

The second treatment option is psychotherapy. Again, this may be in the form of individual, family, or group therapy with a qualified specialist. Cognitive-behavioral therapy is often used.

Chapter 17: Treatments for Associated Disorders

Positive: Some individuals find that discussing their current life issues can greatly reduce their anxiety. Therapists may also assist individuals in facing specific social phobias such as large crowds or public speaking. Family therapy may help each member empathize with the other. Support groups may help the individual relate to others who experience the same disorder.

Negative: Individuals skeptical about therapy may find the treatment very unsatisfying. It may take several sessions for an individual to be able to calm his anxiety. In addition, cognitive-behavioral therapy has a lower success rate with GAD than with other disorders and up to a third of all patients may experience no benefit.[12]

The last treatment option is the act of meditation, relaxation, yoga, or breathing exercises.

Positive: Relaxation exercises can help naturally calm anxiety. An individual may also feel that beginning the day with these rituals could help in staying calmer during daily tasks including working, shopping, and attending events. These techniques may also help provide the individual with more restful sleep.

Negative: Individuals skeptical of these practices may find them less than useful. It may take time to learn various techniques, which may not provide immediate assistance.

6) Posttraumatic Stress Disorder

The first treatment option is medication, which can include SSRIs, antipsychotics, mood stabilizers, antidepressants, or anticonvulsants, depending on the symptoms and the individual.

Chapter 17: Treatments for Associated Disorders

Positive: All of these medications can have positive results. Mood may be elevated and other symptoms of PTSD may be treated simultaneously. Multiple medications may be used to treat different symptoms.

Negative: Different people react differently to medication changes and all of these drugs may have negative side effects including an increase in depression, suicidal ideation, or psychosis. Medication may have only short-term effects if not combined with other treatments. Many of these medications may also create dependence.

The second treatment option is traditional psychotherapy with a qualified specialist in an individual, family, or group setting. Therapists may use verbal or written assignments.

Positive: Discussing or writing about the traumatic experience in a safe environment may prove cathartic. Family therapy may help to resolve issues among members, especially if a family member is the perpetrator. For example, parents may need to cope with an extended family member assaulting their child. Group therapy may provide empathy and support to the victim.

Negative: Some clients may feel that discussing the event will not be beneficial, and will only force them to relive the experience. Ill-trained professionals may not provide adequate tools for healing. Therapy can bring feelings of anger to the surface, which may result in temporary tension in relationships, especially if the anger is misplaced.

The third treatment option is the use of self-help books and workbooks, such as <u>The Courage to Heal</u> by Laura Davis and

Chapter 17: Treatments for Associated Disorders

Ellen Bass. There are also workbooks on the market specifically meant to help treat PTSD.

Positive: Self-help books and workbooks can be an inexpensive tool that may prove very beneficial for some individuals attempting to heal from trauma. These can be used at the person's own pace and inapplicable exercises may be skipped.

Negative: Some individuals may feel that professional help is required, rather than a book. In addition, social interaction may provide assistance that working while isolated will not.

The fourth treatment possibility is the use of Somatic Experiencing. This technique was created by Peter Levine and lets the body and mind heal by released stored energy from the trauma in the nervous system.

Positive: Research has shown that this method can help a person recover from a traumatic event and drastically reduces PTSD symptoms, often the point of elimination with only mild reoccurrence of symptoms. Some individuals may feel that by healing the body and mind simultaneously, they receive more treatment than if they received traditional therapy.

Negative: Individuals skeptical of this method may feel limited results. Specialists certified in Somatic Experiencing may be difficult to locate, especially in rural areas.

The fifth treatment alternative is the attending of workshops. Some clients attend workshops that help them deal with a traumatic event in a group setting with other victims.

Chapter 17: Treatments for Associated Disorders

Positive: Attending workshops may give hands-on training that would be difficult to find in traditional therapy. Individuals may feel additional support from being in a group.

Negative: Workshops of this magnitude can be quite costly. In addition, they may require lengthy travel and the client will be responsible for housing and food costs. Individuals who do not feel comfortable talking about their trauma in a group setting may be very uncomfortable.

The last treatment possibility is exercise and relaxation techniques.

Positive: Exercise can elevate mood, which may reduce some of the PTSD symptoms. Relaxation techniques may allow the person to sleep better or reduce anxiety and hypervigilance.

Negative: Self-motivation can be difficult, especially if exercise is not already a habit. Individuals with medical problems causing chronic pain may have difficulty with moderate to strenuous exercise. Some PTSD victims may find sitting still for an extended period of time, and therefore participating in certain relaxation techniques, very unsettling.

7) Dependent Personality Disorder

Individual and group therapy may be the best tools to assist in DPD.

Positive: Individual therapy may allow a specialist to help a client process aspects of DPD. Group therapy may provide empathy, compassion, and understanding to the struggling individual.

Chapter 17: Treatments for Associated Disorders

Negative: Individuals who are skeptical of treatment may have limited results. Ill-trained professionals may not understand all aspects of the disorder.

8) Avoidant Personality Disorder

Individual and group therapy are important treatment aspects in APD. In addition to traditional therapy, specialists may concentrate on building social skills.

Positive: Individual therapy may provide a safe environment for clients to focus on their social difficulties. Group therapy in addition to specific social skills training may give clients tools to communicate effectively with others.

Negative: Treatment may be difficult, especially in the beginning, and could require excessive practice. This can be frustrating and clients who feel the treatment is ineffective may be unhappy with results. Professionals untrained in proper teaching of social skills may provide only slight benefit to the client.

9) Body Dysmorphic Disorder

The first treatment option is the use of medications, especially SSRIs, which have been discovered to be highly effective.

Positive: Medication may increase positive mood, while decreasing symptoms of BDD.

Negative: SSRIs may carry a risk of dependence. Without the use of other treatment, medication may provide only moderate results.

The second treatment possibility is psychotherapy, especially the use of cognitive-behavioral therapy.

Chapter 17: Treatments for Associated Disorders

Positive: CBT has been proven highly effective in treating BDD.[13] Clients may benefit from discussing their symptoms with a professional in a safe, private setting. Trained professionals can suggest beneficial tools to reduce or eliminate symptoms.

Negative: Clients who are skeptical regarding treatment may find results unsatisfactory. Several sessions may be required to reverse negative thought processes.

10) Dementia

The primary form of treatment for dementia is the use of medications. However, this can vary greatly depending on the cause of dementia.

Positive: Due to the biological causes of dementia, usually from brain or neural abnormalities, medication can be highly effective. Appropriate medication may greatly improve the quality of life for the affected person and for his or her caretakers.

Negative: Some medications can have devastating side effects, including anti-psychotics that are prescribed by medical professionals, although they have not been approved by the Food and Drug Administration (FDA). It has been reported that 2,000 people die in England each year due to the use of these medications.[14] Discuss the possible side effects of any prescribed medications prior to use.

11) Attention Deficit Disorder

The first form of treatment for ADD is medication. Ritalin was the medication that first received outrageous publicity to treat ADHD, and is often still prescribed. However, other medications have also been invented.

Chapter 17: Treatments for Associated Disorders

Positive: Medication has been proven to have positive, short-term effects, including an increase in focus and decrease in distractibility.[15]

Negative: Long-term effects of many of these drugs are still being researched, as is the effectiveness and which medications may wear off with time.[15] In addition, medication for ADHD can be very expensive without insurance, with some pharmacies still charging more than 700 dollars for certain ADD medications.[16]

The second form of treatment is psychotherapy with a specialist usually in an individual setting, but may also be in a family or group setting as well.

Positive: Trained therapists may be able to provide individuals with additional tools to limit distractibility. Clients may find relief in discussing these problems in a safe environment. Family therapy will allow each member to express him or herself and provide tools to minimize the effects of ADD. Group therapy may provide support and new ideas to those struggling.

Negative: Individuals skeptical of treatment may find minimal benefits. If the impairment is biological, rather than psychological or behavioral, therapy may have limited results without the use of medication.

The third treatment option is intense hands-on training. Several states now have summer programs available for ADD and ADHD children, in which they learn additional social and cognitive skills, receive schooling assistance, and meet others who are also struggling with these disorders. These programs may last between two and twelve weeks, depending on the program and curriculum.

Chapter 17: Treatments for Associated Disorders

Positive: Some of these programs have been highly successful.[17] Children may return to school and home with a new perspective and improved methods for daily activities, learning, and building peer relationships. Financial assistance may be provided to individuals and families with limited income.

Negative: Some of these programs, especially extensive programs, can be very costly. Because many states still do not have these programs, families may have to drive or fly to a different part of the country. If children do not want to participate, they may experience limited benefits.

The fourth treatment option is a change in diet and exercise such as lowering the intake of sugary foods.

Positive: Allowing individuals with ADD or ADHD time to be active may increase mood and later increase focus. The reduction of sugar may also decrease distractibility and hyper movements. ADD individuals may enjoy exercise, and motivation may not be as much of a problem as it would be for depressed individuals.

Negative: Motivation may be difficult, especially if the person's current diet has a large amount of sugar. Exercise may pose difficult for individuals in chronic pain.

Note: Caffeine generally calms individuals with ADD/ADHD. This is due to caffeine being a stimulant, which is also the type of medication that is prescribed. Although caffeine may make an individual without ADD *more* hyper, it often has the opposite effect on true ADD/ADHD individuals. Drinking coffee without sugar may help an individual focus at school or work, especially if the caffeine drinking occurs throughout the day.

Chapter 17: Treatments for Associated Disorders

12) Diogenes Syndrome

Lifestyle changes are the primary form of treatment for this disorder. Lifestyle changes include interventions for hoarding, exposure to social interaction (which may include the teaching of social skills), improvement in self-care, and possible placement in a senior care center.

Positive: Lifestyle changes and outside interventions may have great benefits in some or all symptoms. In addition, these changes may improve quality of life for the affected person and their family members and caregivers.

Negative: These changes may be very difficult, especially in individuals who do not believe there is a problem. Initial attempts may be very time-consuming by others with minimal results. Professional assistance may be required, which can be quite costly.

Often, OCD and compulsive hoarding must be treated in addition to other present disorders, such as those listed above.

Chapter 17: Treatments for Associated Disorders

Notes

1. American Psychiatric Association. (2000). Practice guideline for the treatment of patients with major depressive disorder. *American Journal of Psychiatry.* 157(Supp 4), 1-45.

2. Sackeim, H. A., Haskett, R. F., and Mulsant, B. H. (2001). Continuation pharmacotherapy in the prevention of relapse following electroconvulsive therapy: A randomized controlled trial. *Journal of the American Medical Association. 285(10),* 1299-1307.

3. Poolsup, N., Li Wan Po, A., and De Oliveira, I. R. (2000). Systematic overview of lithium treatment in acute mania. *Journal of clinical pharmacy and therapeutics. 25(2),* 139–156.

4. Geddes, J. R., Burgess, S., Hawton, K., Jamison, K., and Goodwin, G. M. (2004). Long-term lithium therapy for bipolar disorder: Systematic review and meta-analysis of randomized controlled trials. *The American Journal of Psychiatry. 161(2),* 217–222.

5. Geddes, J. R., Calabrese, J. R., and Goodwin, G. M. (2008). Lamotrigine for treatment of bipolar depression: Independent meta-analysis and meta-regression of individual patient data from five randomized trials. *The British Journal of Psychiatry. 194(1),* 4–9.

6. Van Der Loos, M. L., Kölling, P., Knoppert-Van Der Klein, E. A, and Nolen, W. A. (2007). Lamotrigine in the treatment of bipolar disorder, a review. *Tijdschrift voor psychiatrie. 49(2),* 95–103.

Chapter 17: Treatments for Associated Disorders

7. Westenberg, HG. (Jul 1999). "Facing the challenge of social anxiety disorder". *Eur Neuropsychopharmacol.* 9(Suppl 3), S93–9.

8. Barlow, D. H., Gorman, J. M., Shear, M. K., and Woods, S. W. (May 2000). "Cognitive-behavioral therapy. *Journal of the American Medical Association. 283(19),* 2529–2536.

9. Marks, I. M., Swinson, R.P., Başoğlu M., *et al.* (June 1993). Alprazolam and exposure alone and combined in panic disorder with agoraphobia: A controlled study in London and Toronto. *British Journal of Psychiatry. 162(6),* 776–787.

10. Choy, Y. (2008). Treatment Planning for Panic Disorder. *Psychiatric Times. 25(2).*

11. Stewart, S.H., and Westrac H.A. (2002). Benzodiazepine side-effects: from the bench to the clinic. *Curr. Pharm. Des. 8(1),* 1–3.

12. Barlow, D. H. (2007). *Clinical Handbook of Psychological Disorders*, 4th ed.

13. Rosen, J. C., Reiter, J., Orosan, P. (1995). Cognitive-behavioral body image therapy for body dysmorphic disorder. *Journal of Consulting and Clinical Psychology. 63(2),* 263–269.

14. Bowcott, O. (Nov. 12, 2009). Chemical restraints killing dementia. London: Guardian. http://www.guardian.co.uk/society/2009/nov/12/anti-psychotic-drugs-kill-dementia-patients.

15. Butcher, J.N., Mineka, S., & Hooley, J. M. (2010). *Abnormal psychology.* (14th ed.). Boston: Allyn & Bacon. pp. 530-533.

Chapter 17: Treatments for Associated Disorders

16. Various observations and interviews.

17. Mash, E. J. & Wolfe, D. A. (2010). Abnormal child psychology. (4th ed.) Belmont, CA: Wadsworth.

Chapter 18: What Does Future Research Look Like?

Various research has been discussed throughout this book. However, new research is always being conducted and the future holds endless possibilities in diagnosis and treatment. This chapter will examine the possibilities of new treatments.

Can we expect new treatments? Absolutely. The amount of information regarding these disorders and the brain has increased exceptionally in the past three decades due to technological advances. These advances are continuing and brain imaging is become much more detailed. There are currently new brain imaging techniques being tested that will give a clearer picture of which parts of the brain manage which behaviors. As new images are created, a more in depth understanding of causes occur, the more treatment options including medications, and possibly non-invasive surgery, can occur.

With the possible addition of hoarding as a separate disorder to the DSM-V, more therapists and psychiatrists may become aware of the problem, how to diagnose it, and ways to treat it. Professionals having a wider understanding may ensure that your friend or family member receives superb care from anyone they choose to see.

New medications are being tested all the time. As new developments occur with brain and genetic abnormalities, new medications may become available to target specific chemicals, areas of the brain, neurotransmitters, and genes.

Although alternative, holistic medication has been used for centuries, there may be new developments based on research regarding the causes of these disorders.

Chapter 18: What does Future Research Look Like?

Even if the treatment this person is receiving right now does not seem to be helping, encourage them to continue to experiment with new forms of medication, therapy, and holistic medicine. The future should give additional hope of improved treatment options.

Chapter 19: A Special Look at Children

Children and adolescents can also receive a diagnosis of OCD, but these age groups may have different characteristics from each other and from their adult counterparts.

Some researchers state that the typical age of onset for OCD is late adolescence and early adulthood, although it is also common in children.[1] Others say that the average age of onset is between 9 and 12 years of age.[2] Research also differs regarding how similar the symptoms may be between children and adults.

For the purpose of this book, simply understand that it is not an uncommon disorder for children and adolescents and research shows that there are some differences in the disorder among age groups, which will be discussed here.

As many as two to three percent of children and adolescents may suffer from OCD and, although statistics vary, up to two-thirds of these children may still have symptoms up to 14 years later.[2]

Individuals who develop OCD prior to age 11, often have a family history of the disorder. This may be evidence of a greater genetic linkage, as discussed in previous chapters.[2]

Children may have the same obsessions and compulsions as their adult counterparts including the need for symmetry, checking, and repetitive behaviors. In addition, children are often most fearful of germs and others being harmed.[2]

To an extent, it is normal for a child to fear loved ones becoming injured or dying, especially children who have only recently learned about death. However, again, this fear becomes a disorder when functionality is impaired. If a child seems constantly distressed at these thoughts, you may consider seeking treatment.

For children, other disorders associated with OCD include learning disorders, eating disorders, and substance abuse

Chapter 19: A Special Look at Children

disorders.[2] Substance abuse may begin as a coping skill for adolescents to help numb or minimize the obsessions. However, this coping skill is harmful and not a permanent or healthy treatment.

Some research shows that boys may be more likely to be diagnosed with OCD than girls.[2] However, this bias may be more due to boys being referred for mental health services more often, especially due to acting out behaviors, and therefore are more frequently diagnosed.

Treatments of OCD in children and adolescents are similar to those of adults. Children may benefit greatly from therapy or alternative medicine. However, some medications that are used on adults may be dangerous to be given to children and adolescents. Research medication and talk to your primary care physician or psychiatrist prior to starting your child's prescription.

It is rare for children to develop hoarding behaviors, which are most often not developed until at least adolescence.[3] If your child does hoard, refer to treatments used in hoarding behaviors in adults.

As you can see, children and adolescents differ from adults in some specific ways, although the overall symptoms are very similar. It is helpful to know that treatments are available, even for children at a young age.

Chapter 19: A Special Look at Children

Notes

1. Butcher, J.N., Mineka, S., & Hooley, J. M. (2010). *Abnormal psychology.* (14th ed.). Boston: Allyn & Bacon. pp. 206-216.

2. Mash, E. J. & Wolfe, D. A. (2010). Abnormal child psychology. (4th ed.) Belmont, CA: Wadsworth. pp. 206-209.

3. Bratiotis, C., Otte, S., Steketee, G., Muroff, J., & Frost, R. O. International OCD Foundation. (2009). Hoarding Fact Sheet. Retrieved from http://www.ocfoundation.org/uploadedFiles/Hoarding%20Fact%20Sheet.pdf?n=3557.

Chapter 20: Living with a Person with OCD

Whether this person has decided to seek treatment, you remain living with him or her and this relationship may become strained. Here is a list of tips you may be able to use to make living with this person more enjoyable.

1) You may recommend the individual seek treatment. Refer to previous chapters for guidance.
2) If the person makes any improvement, no matter how slight, take notice. As stated earlier, symptoms of OCD can increase and decrease gradually. If symptoms have decreased or seem to be in remission, bring this to the person's attention. Do not be patronizing or condescending, as this will only result in the person becoming defensive, embarrassed, and hurt.
3) You may want to keep a note of compulsions in which you notice the person engaging. This may be too difficult or painful for the person to do for him or herself. This information may be helpful in finding a pattern for the OCD; which symptoms are improving or getting worse, and what to tell therapists or medical professionals.
4) Understand that this is a disorder that may be causing the person a great amount of anxiety. Be supportive and listen if the person decides to discuss their struggle.
5) Follow any recommendations a therapist or psychiatrist has given.
6) If the OCD is so severe that it is obvious to strangers, warn anyone you will bring home, prior to introducing them. This will give the other person time to adjust and may

Chapter 20: Living with a Person with OCD

make it a smoother transition for the person with OCD, reducing anxiety.
7) Understand that we all have our burdens and you may also have behaviors or characteristics that others must learn to tolerate.

Although living with someone with OCD may pose serious strain on your relationship, try to see the other person's perspective and be understanding of their struggle.

Chapter 21: Living with a Person who Hoards

An individual who hoards can be difficult to live with, especially if you are a person who is considered neat and orderly.

1) You may recommend the individual seek treatment. Refer to previous chapters for guidance.
2) If the person makes any improvement, no matter how slight, take notice. This may include something that you consider small such as throwing away the junk mail from the kitchen counter. The person may have struggled with this decision while you weren't there. It's important to provide positive reinforcement, so that the positive behavior may continue in the future.
3) Attempt to limit the hoarding to a room or area of the room, such as a garage or closet. The more confined the disorganized mess is, the less anxiety that will occur, seeing as it will not have as many negative effects on the living situation.
4) Understand that this is a disorder that may be causing the person a great amount of anxiety. Be supportive and listen if the person decides to discuss their struggle.
5) If the person wants to clean or organize, offer to help. It may seem less overwhelming if there is at least one other person assisting. However, be careful as to what you throw away and you may need to ask before you toss anything, no matter how small.

Chapter 21: Living with a Person who Hoards

6) Don't bring home company unexpectedly. This may cause embarrassment, anger, and anxiety from the person who

hoards due to the mess not being presentable, at least to this person. Give them plenty of time to tidy up. Several days or more is preferable. You may also avoid this in entirely by meeting in a different location.
7) If the person hoards food, arrange for the person to keep a small box or container of food in their room. This food should be non-perishable and have no restrictions. Often, hoarders will not eat the food, they simply want to know that it is accessible. If the food is eaten, or if it eventually goes bad, replace it. Foods to consider are canned goods, nuts, crackers, and even peanut butter if it has not yet been open. Do not use any food or packaging that could attract insects or rodents.
8) Understand that we all have our burdens and you may also have behaviors or characteristics that others must learn to tolerate.

Although living with someone who hoards may pose serious strain on your relationship, try to see the other person's perspective and be understanding of their struggle.

Chapter 22: Working with a Person with OCD

Although you may not be living with this person, an individual suffering from OCD may also pose challenges to coworkers and the work environment. Here are some tips to hopefully make the relationship easier.

1) Unless you know the person well, do not attempt to persuade them to seek treatment or act as if you are diagnosing them. This will most likely only lead to defensive behavior.
2) Realize that unless the person has confided in you, you probably won't know if the person has already sought treatment. They may already be in therapy and be trying to do better.
3) Find positive aspects of the disorder and brag on those characteristics. Maybe this person is always prepared for important meetings because they read the literature three times prior to attending. Focus a positive light on the fact that the individual is prepared, but do not bring up the compulsion, as this may only embarrass, anger, or exhaust the individual.
4) Understand that we all have our burdens and you may also have behaviors or characteristics that others must learn to tolerate.

Provide an empathetic and supportive ear. After strengthening the relationship, your coworker may appreciate being able to talk to someone about their struggles. If they do, make sure you communicate that you understand this is a treatable disorder, not an annoying personality trait.

Chapter 23: Working with a Person who Hoards

A person who hoards may make for a disorganized coworker. Working with this person may pose certain challenges. Here are some tips to hopefully make this relationship easier on both of you.

1) Unless you know this person well, don't suggest treatment. Most likely, the person would only become defensive, furthering the tension in your relationship.
2) Realize that unless the person has confided in you, you probably won't know if the person has already sought treatment. They may already be in therapy and be trying to do better.
3) Try to keep workspaces separate. As long as your space is uncluttered, attempt to accept the mess in the other person's space.
4) If the office is straightened or cleaned one day, be positive. "Wow, it looks really good in here." Don't be condescending or patronizing as this will only make the person angry and defensive.
5) Understand that we all have our burdens and you may also have behaviors or characteristics that others must learn to tolerate.

In conclusion, try to understand your coworker's struggle and realize that this behavior is part of a disorder that can cause great anxiety. Being kind and empathetic may improve the relationship without any additional assistance.

Chapter 24: Additional Resources Available

Although this book has hopefully helped you immensely, you may want to seek additional resources as well. This chapter will list websites and organizations that will hopefully help you as well.

1) Hoarding

Films
- Grey Gardens (Director: Ellen Hoyde, etc.)
- Information about Compulsive Hoarding (with Dr. Renae M. Reinardy)
- My Mother's Garden (Director: Cynthia Lester)
- Packrat (Director: Kris Britt Montag)
- Stuffed (Director: Arwen Curry and Cerissa Tanner)

Books
- Buried in Treasures: Help for Compulsive Acquiring, Saving, and Hoarding by David F. Tolin, Robert O. Frost, and Gail Steketee ISBN: 978-0195300581
- Digging Out: Helping Your Loved One Manage Clutter, Hoarding, and Compulsive Acquiring by Michael A. Thompkins and Tamara L. Hartl ISBN: 978-1572245945
- Overcoming Compulsive Hoarding: Why You Save and How You Can Stop by Jerome Bubrick, Fugen Neziroglu, and Jose Yarvura-Tobias
ISBN: 978-1572243491

Chapter 24: Additional Resources Available

- Stuff: Compulsive Hoarding and the Meaning of Things by Robert O. Frost and Gail Steketee ISBN: 978-0151014231

Organizations
International Obsessive Compulsive Disorder Foundation
www.ocdfoundation.org

Institute for Challenging Disorganization
www.challengingdisorganization.org

National Association of Professional Organizers
Website: http://www.napo.net

The Compulsive Hoarding Center
www.compulsivehoardingcenter.com

Support Groups

Listing of Community Hoarding Task Forces
Website: http://www.hoardingtaskforce.com

Clutterers Anonymous
Website: http://www.clutterersanonymous.net

Messies Anonymous
Website: http://www.messies.com

Chapter 24: Additional Resources Available

2) Obsessive Compulsive Disorder

Books
Overcoming Obsessive-Compulsive Disorder: A Self-Help Guide Using Cognitive Behavioral Techniques by David Veale and Robert Wilson
ISBN: 978-0465011087

Mobile Apps
Live OCD Free

Organizations
International Obsessive Compulsive Disorder Foundation
www.ocdfoundation.org

3) For Children and Teens

Books
- A Thought is Just a Thought: A Story of Living with OCD by Leslie Talley ISBN: 978-1590560655
- Blink, Blink, Clop, Clop: Why Do We Do Things We Can't Stop? An OCD Storybook by E. Katia Moritz and Jennifer Jablonsky ISBN: 978-1882732722
- Mr. Worry: A Story about OCD by Holly L. Niner ISBN: 978-0807551820
- No One is Perfect and YOU Are a Great Kid by Kim Hix ISBN: 978-1419631481

Chapter 24: Additional Resources Available

- Not as Crazy as I Seem by George Harrar ISBN: 978-0618494804 Take Control of OCD: The Ultimate Guide for Kids with OCD by Bonnie Zucker ISBN: 978-1593634292
- Talking Back to OCD: The Program That Helps Kids and Teens to Say "No Way"—and Parents to Say "Way to Go" by John S. March ISBN: 978-1593853556
- The Ray of Hope: A Teenager's Fight Against Obsessive Compulsive Disorder by Ray St John ISBN: 978-0578070322
- Up and Down the Worry Hill: A Children's Book about Obsessive Compulsive Disorder and Its Treatment by Aureen Pinto Wagner and Paul A. Justton ISBN: 978-0967734767
- What to Do When Your Brain Gets Stuck: A Kid's Guide to Overcoming OCD by Dawn Huebner ISBN: 978-1591478058
- You Do That Too? by Rena Benson and Jose Arturo ISBN: 978-0963907059

4) For Parents

Books
- Freeing Your Child From Obsessive-Compulsive Disorder: A Powerful, Practical Program for Parents of Children and Adolescents by Tamar E. Chansky ISBN: 978-0812931174
- Helping Your Child with OCD: A Workbook for Parents of Children with Obsessive- Compulsive Disorder by Lee Fitzgibbons and Cherlene Pedrick ISBN: 978-1572243323
- Obsessive-Compulsive Disorder: Helping Children and Adolescents by Mitzi Waltz ISBN: 978-1565927582

Chapter 24: Additional Resources Available

- Talking Back to OCD: The Program That Helps Kids and Teens to Say "No Way"—and Parents to Say "Way to Go" by John S. March ISBN: 978-1593853556
- What To Do When Your Child Has Obsessive-Compulsive Disorder: Strategies and Solutions by Aureen Pinto Wagner ISBN: 978-0967734712

5) For Teachers

Film
OCD in the Classroom: A Multi-Media Program for Parents, Teachers, and School Personnel by Marlene Targ Brill and Gail B. Adams

6) Treatments

Materials
Treatment of OCD in Children and Adolescents: Professional's Kit

Organizations
Association for Behavioral and Cognitive Therapies
www.abct.org

National Association of Professional Organizers
www.napo.net

Chapter 24: Additional Resources Available

American Academy of Child and Adolescent Psychiatry
Website: http://www.aacap.org

Anxiety Disorders Association of America
Website: http://www.adaa.org

Awareness Foundation for OCD
Website: http://www.afocd.org

Beyond OCD
website: www.beyondocd.org

Clutterers Anonymous
Website: http://www.clutterersanonymous.net

Freedom From Fear
Website: http://www.freedomfromfear.org

National Alliance on Mental Illness
Website: http://www.nami.org

National Disability Rights Network
Website: http://www.ndrn.org

Obsessive Compulsive Anonymous (OCA)
Website: http://obsessivecompulsiveanonymous.org

The OCD Challenge
Website: http://www.ocdchallenge.com

Chapter 24: Additional Resources Available

OCD Education Station

Website: http://www.ocdeducationstation.org

The Other OCD: "Purely-Obsessional" OCD
Website: www.theotherocd.com

Relief Resources
Website: http://www.reliefhelp.org

7) Children of Hoarders

Books
- Keepsake: A Novel by Kristina Riggle ISBN: 978-0062003072
Nice Children Stolen from Car by Barbara K Allen ISBN: 978-1475192636
- Never Say Sorry by Rose Edmunds (Kindle Format)
Dirty Secret: A Daughter Comes Clean About Her Mother's Compulsive Hoarding ISBN: 1439192529
- Dirty Little Secrets by C.J. Omololu ISBN: 978-0802722331
- Where the Sun Don't Shine and the Shadows Don't Play: Growing Up with an   Obsessive Compulsive Hoarder ISBN: 978-1462034475

Organizations
Children of Hoarders™

www.childrenofhoarders.com

Support Groups
List of In-Person Support Groups by State
www. http://childrenofhoarders.com/wordpress/?page_id=4318

Chapter 24: Additional Resources Available

Online Support Group
 Yahoo! Groups: children of hoarders
http://health.groups.yahoo.com/group/childrenofhoarders/

8) Financial Assistance
Organizations:

For Treatment:

Anxiety Disorders Foundation
Website: http://www.anxietydisordersfoundation.org

For Prescriptions:

Needy Meds
Website: http://www.needymeds.org

Partnership for Prescription Assistance
Website: http://www.pparx.org

For Insurance:

Cover the Uninsured
Website: http://covertheuninsured.org

Medicare Rights Center
Website: http://www.medicarerights.org
Anxiety Disorders Association of America
Website: http://www.adaa.org

Association for Behavioral and Cognitive Therapies
Website: http://www.abct.org

Chapter 24: Additional Resources Available

9) Legal Resources and Employment Assistance
Organizations

Americans with Disabilities Act
U.S. Department of Justice
Website: http://www.ada.gov

Individuals with Disabilities Act (IDEA)
Website: http://idea.ed.gov

Office of Disability Employment Policy
U.S. Department of Labor
Website: http://www.dol.gov/odep

Chapter 25: Conclusion

OCD and hoarding are both disorders that can have severe negative effects on the afflicted individual as well as people around him or her. However, treatments are available to assist in minimizing these effects.

Learning information about a disorder can make it easier for a person to understand a person diagnosed with it. This can extend to living with or working with the person. Hopefully, gaining this knowledge has helped you to tolerate behaviors you may have believed to be intentional.

Although research has come a long way in the past few decades, additional research is still needed, especially in the area of brain imaging and medication management. Seeking treatment and choosing the right treatment for each case is a personal decision that should not be taken lightly.

Hopefully, this book has helped many people. Make the most of your life, regardless of the disorders you or a loved one may be diagnosed with. Each of us chooses our own destiny.

Glossary

Agoraphobia—the fear of large crowds.

Alzheimer's Disease—a neurological disorder that results in severe brain abnormalities which cause memory loss, impaired cognitive functioning, and deterioration of motor skills.

Attention Deficit Disorder (ADD)—a mental health disorder characterized by an inability to concentrate with thought processes quickly changing, which may result in memory problems.

Avoidant personality disorder (APD) –a mental health disorder characterized by a fear of criticism that causes the person to avoid social situations, although they still desire affection and attention.

Bipolar Disorder (BPD)—a disorder in which, part of the time the patient is manic and at other points may be extremely depressed.

Body dysmorphic disorder—a mental health disorder in which a person is obsessed with her or her body, or a part of the body.

Dementia—a disorder characterized by a decrease in functioning, especially in memory and the ability to process information.

Dependent personality disorder (DPD) –a mental health disorder characterized by a need to be taken care of due to feelings of being inept when alone.

Flashback—an occurrence similar to a memory in which the individual feels that he or she is reliving the traumatic experience.

Glossary

Formication (tactile hallucinations)—the feeling that insects are crawling on or under the skin, despite the fact that there is no physical evidence.

Generalized anxiety disorder (GAD)—a mental health disorder in which a person almost always feels a sense of anxiety.

Hoarding-- continuing to hold possessions after their intended use has ended.

Human Immunodeficiency Virus (HIV)—a blood condition which drastically weakens the immune system and eventually leads to acquired immune deficiency syndrome (AIDS) and death.

Huntington's Disease—a disease that affects the central nervous system and results in spontaneous, involuntary motions that begin in one area of the body and spread.

Hypervigilance—the state of being overly aware.

Hypomania—a state of lessened mania in which some symptoms are present, but are not yet severe.

Mania—a state of extreme hyperactivity in which a person may be unable to think or behave logically.

Neurotransmitter—an area of nerves that send signals to other nerves to transmit messages and follow-up actions.

Obsessive-Compulsive Disorder (OCD)—a mental health problem that includes thoughts and behaviors that are intrusive, redundant, anal, or habitual, usually against the control of the afflicted person impeding his or her function.

Glossary

Panic disorder—a mental health disorder in which panic attacks are frequent and seem to have no particular onset.

Parkinson's Disease—a disorder in which a loss of dopamine neurons in specific parts of the brain will result in the body having tremors and spontaneous movements.

Psychiatrist—a mental health professional who has received a medical degree (MD) and can prescribe psychiatric medication.

Prevalence—how common a disorder is, and in which demographics it is more likely to occur.

Social Anxiety—a feeling of distress upon entering social situations.

Social phobia—an intense fear of specific social situations such as public speaking, eating in public, or being surrounded by too many people.

Socioeconomic status (SES)—an individual, or family's, income, education, profession, and residence.

Stroke—a neurological malfunction that occurs when the brain does not receive enough blood, and therefore oxygen, which results in brain damage.

Therapist—a mental health professional who has received training in diagnosing and treating various mental disorders.

Vascular Dementia—a disorder that has symptoms similar to Alzheimer's disease but is due to blood being lost to specific areas of the brain for a short period of time.

Index

Index

ADD. See Attention deficit disorder
ADHD. See Attention deficit disorder
Alternative medicine, 111, 116, 153
Alzheimer's disease, 89, 90, 91, 178
Animal Hoarding, 27
APD. See Avoidant Personality Disorder
Attention Deficit Disorder, 3, 4, 93, 142, 175
Avoidant Personality Disorder, 4, 78 140
BDD. See Body Dysmorphic Disorder
Bipolar Disorder, 4, 83 126, 175
Body Dysmorphic Disorder, 2, 4, 79, 141 149
Book Hoarding, 31
BPD. See Bipolar Disorder
Checking, 49
Cognitive-behavioral therapy, 112, 123, 127, 131, 133, 135, 148
Combined Obsessive and Compulsive Type, 23
Compulsive Hoarding. See Hoarding
Counting, 51
Dementia, 3, 4, 66, 88, 89, 90, 92, 106, 141, 142, 149, 175, 178
Dependent Personality Disorder, 4, 78, 139
Digital Hoarding, 29
Diogenes Syndrome, 3, 4, 29, 94, 106, 145
DPD. See Dependent Personality Disorder
Fear of Causing Harm to Others, 53
Fear of Contamination (Cleaning), 48
GAD. See Generalized Anxiety Disorder
Generalized Anxiety Disorder, 4, 73, 134
HIV. See Human Immunodeficiency Virus
Hoarding, 1-3, 5-6, 13-14, 16-17, 20, 27-31, 33-34, 38-42, 58, 60-62, 64-69, 82-83, 85-88, 92-96, 102, 104-106, 108-109, 112, 115,-116, 145-146, 150, 153, 155, 158, 164, 165, 171, 174, 176
Human Immunodeficiency Virus, 92, 176
Huntington's disease, 89, 90
Information Hoarding, 31
Lifestyle changes, 111, 112, 116, 118
Major Depressive Disorder, 2, 4, 72, 122
MDD. See Major Depressive Disorder

Index

Medication, 3, 46, 111, 116, 136, 141-142
Obsessive compulsive disorder, 9, 115, 121
OCD. See Obsessive Compulsive Disorder
Other Obsessions and Compulsions, 58
Panic attacks, 74, 133, 177
Panic disorder, 73, 74, 75, 132, 148
Parkinson's disease, 89, 90
Posttraumatic Stress Disorder, 4, 73 86, 136
Psychotherapy, 111, 116, 117, 123, 124, 127, 128, 131, 132, 135, 137, 141, 143

PTSD. See Posttraumatic Stress Disorder
Purely Obsessive Type, 23
Religious Obsessions, 56
Repetitive Behaviors, 52
Rituals, 57
Sexual Obsessions, 56
Social anxiety, 86, 130, 148
Social phobia, 73, 74, 86, 130
Surgery, 111, 114, 150
Syllogomania. See Trash Hoarding
Symmetry, 55
Trash Hoarding, 29
Vascular dementia, 91

CPSIA information can be obtained at www.ICGtesting.com
Printed in the USA
LVOW121656170513

334354LV00024B/724/P